# Problem-based Learning for Health Improvement

## Practical public health for every professional

T0133916

### Edited by

## John Cornell

*Director of Public Health*
*Doncaster Central Primary Care Trust*

## and

## Frada Eskin

*Consultant in Public Health Medicine*
*Sheffield Health Authority*

### Foreword by

## Professor Sir Liam Donaldson

*Chief Medical Officer*
*England*

Radcliffe Medical Press

**Radcliffe Medical Press Ltd**
18 Marcham Road
Abingdon
Oxon OX14 1AA
United Kingdom


**www.radcliffe-oxford.com**
The Radcliffe Medical Press electronic catalogue and online ordering facility.
Direct sales to anywhere in the world.

---

British Library Cataloguing in Publication Data

A catalogue record for this book is available from the British Library.

ISBN 1 85775 501 4

Typeset by Advance Typesetting Ltd, Oxfordshire
Printed and bound by TJ International Ltd, Padstow, Cornwall

# Contents

# Foreword

Some years ago I was in a meeting discussing a proposed programme of organisational development in the NHS. The challenge for the morning was, amongst other things, to come up with a name for the programme which would both inspire and motivate staff and communicate a clear sense of purpose. Inevitably someone suggested 'Making it happen'. Such was the groundswell of support for this heart-sinking idea that in an attempt to head it off I argued for the need for some originality rather than yet again plagiarising John Harvey-Jones's catch-phrase. Confronted with having to put up or shut up and desperate to inject some humour into a very dull meeting and given that the initiative was to be based partly in Yorkshire, I suggested ' 'appen it'll 'appen'. Regrettably, the idea was initially taken seriously but later dropped in favour of something with a Shakespearean evocation.

When I read *Problem-based Learning for Health Improvement* I reflected on how many times over the last few decades public health has been challenged with developing its role in a newly reorganised NHS. The emphasis in the past has been too much on the laissez-faire and not enough on actively seeking to shape the future.

The beginning of the 21st century has brought a positive context for public health practice in the United Kingdom which is unparalleled. A new focus for delivery through public health teams in primary care, a fresh impetus to multi-professional practice, a wide range of cross government policies directed at health improvement, a repositioning of health protection centre stage, the health strand being added to other regeneration programmes, and the reduction of health inequalities finally being declared as a national priority.

This is a climate which demands a positive and proactive response from the public health community. This new text is an important part of the endeavour to 'make it happen'. Practical, problem-orientated and insightful, each chapter addresses one of the 10 areas of public health competency defined by the Faculty of Public Health Medicine of the Royal College of Physicians.

The project was led by its editor Dr Frada Eskin, the innovative public health thinker and teacher known and loved by generations of public health trainees.

The book deserves to be well read but, more importantly, well used by all those who are committed to achieving real improvement in the health of local communities.

**Sir Liam Donaldson**
**Chief Medical Officer**
*January 2003*

# About the authors

**Tony Baxter** is Director of Public Health for Doncaster East Primary Care Trust. He is passionate about training and has been an examiner for the UK Faculty of Public Health since 1999.

**John Cornell** qualified in Manchester in 1975. After training in surgery, he trained in general practice and became a principal in Sheffield in 1984. He entered public health in 1994 and was appointed Consultant in Public Health Medicine in Doncaster in 1998. He was appointed as Director of Public Health to Doncaster Central Primary Care Trust (PCT) in 2002. His main areas of activity are implementing locally the Coronary Heart Disease National Framework, Caldicott implementation in primary care and developing the public health functions of the PCT.

**Frances Cunning** has been working in health promotion since 1986, first as a health promotion specialist in Cumbria, then as Deputy Director of Health Promotion in Sheffield. Prior to her current role as Head of Sheffield's Strategic Health Partnership Support Unit, Frances was Assistant Director of Policy and Public Health in Sheffield.

**Frada Eskin** qualified in medicine at the University of Sheffield in 1960. She chose to make her medical career in the field of public health. After being appointed to various posts in public health in Sheffield and in Derbyshire, she left public health practice in 1975 to run a Department of Health-funded National Continuing Education Unit based in the Department of Social and Preventive Medicine in the medical school at Manchester University, where she spent the next 14 years as director of the unit. During this time she developed expertise in management education and personal development, which she was able to integrate into public health medicine training. She returned to work in the NHS in 1989 as consultant in public health medicine at Yorkshire Health and then as Deputy Director of Public Health for Sheffield Health Authority, from where she retired in July 2001. She has published widely on a variety of public health topics, management and personal development, including two books and a substantial number of papers.

**Paul Fryers** has degrees in statistics from St Andrew's University and public health from the Nuffield Institute in Leeds. He has worked in the NHS within the Yorkshire and Humber region for 11 years and is currently head of the Public Health Intelligence Unit in Doncaster.

**Elizabeth Goyder** is a clinical lecturer in public health in the School of Health and Related Research (ScHARR) at the University of Sheffield. Prior to this she was involved in public health research in Mumbai (India), Sydney (Australia) and Leicester (UK). In her current post, as well as teaching public health to medical students, she has worked for North Derbyshire Health Authority, the Trent Public Health Observatory and the policy branch of the Department of Health. Her current public health research interests include inequalities in health and access to health services, particularly in relation to type 2 diabetes and screening for type 2 diabetes. In 2002 she received a national Public Health Career Scientist Award for this research programme.

**Rosy McNaught** qualified in Sheffield in 1979 and, after initial hospital posts, trained in public health in the Northern region. She has been the Consultant in Communicable Disease Control for Sheffield since 1992 where she has a special interest in infectious diseases and emergency planning.

**James Munro** is consultant senior lecturer in epidemiology at the Medical Care Research Unit, University of Sheffield. His clinical background is in hospital general medicine and public health medicine. Current research interests include the effects of the new UK immediate care services, patient removals by GPs, pre-operative testing, physical activity in older adults and British health policy generally. He is the founding editor of *Health Matters*, an independent quarterly magazine on health policy and politics, public health advisor to the Centre for Innovation in Primary Care and co-editor of *Promoting Health: politics and practice, Healthy Choices: future options for the NHS* and *The Evidence-based Medicine Workbook*.

**Angela Scott** originally qualified as a science teacher and taught secondary and further education pupils. Angela then moved into health promotion, working initially with schools, before being appointed as Director of Health Promotion. Angela is currently working as Associate Director of Health Policy and Public Health and is the designated Teenage Pregnancy Co-ordinator and the HAZ-wide Children and Young People Programme Area Lead for the South Yorkshire Coalfields Health Action Zone (HAZ).

**Darren Shickle** is a clinical senior lecturer in public health medicine at the University of Sheffield and an honorary consultant at North Eastern Derbyshire Primary Care Trust. He was previously a 1996–97 Harkness Fellow at the Bioethics Institute, Johns Hopkins University, Baltimore, USA. His research interests are public health ethics and genetics.

**Ian Welborn** is a chartered occupational psychologist and an independent management consultant with extensive experience of working in the NHS over the last 15 years. He has worked very closely with public health during this period, with a particular interest in leadership development, team development, communications and interpersonal skill development, trainer development and the management of change.

# Introduction

*Frada Eskin and John Cornell*

## Developing a public health perspective

Improving the health of the population requires a public health perspective. We have written this book to demonstrate its nature. Improving the population's health is the occupational *raison d'être* of public health professionals. However, because the population's health is affected by all facets of society's activities (*see* Figure A), possessing a public health perspective is relevant to a wide variety of other professions and disciplines. Although doctors and nurses, social workers, teachers, etc., work with individuals, this book provides new insights for them to consider individuals within the wider context and offers increased possibilities for problem solving. For example, poor living conditions adversely affect school-work, dysfunctional families militate against a patient's recovery and fear of violence on a housing estate limits the social life of an older person, which in turn creates isolation, loneliness and health deterioration. Given this broader perspective, the solution to a problem may lie in improving the wider environment rather than focusing on the symptoms exhibited by the individual. Taking a public health perspective therefore increases the opportunities for improving the population's health and well-being.

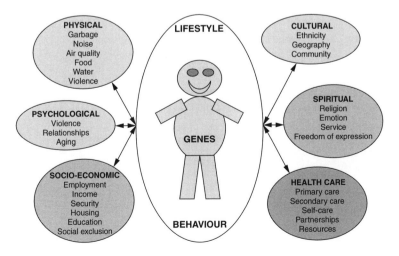

**Figure A:**　Friend or foe? The environment and its effect on health.

We aim to demonstrate to readers, through practical examples, the network of knowledge and skills required to tackle the challenges that daily confront all professionals concerned with people's health. Each chapter is devoted to exploring one of the ten areas of public health competence as defined by the Faculty of Public Health Medicine.[1] This has been achieved using a problem-based, self-directed learning model. Each of the chapter authors was given a broad brief but with some leeway and licence in how they presented their work. This reflects the reality of public health practice.

Every chapter in this book is a discrete entity and can be studied without reference to any other chapter. However, because public health comprises an intricately interwoven set of competencies, the reader is warned that to take one chapter on its own does not always enable a view of the full picture.

Where relevant, we have cross-referenced to other chapters, illustrating connected themes and avoiding duplication. The book is, of itself, a learning experience. It is a journey, which, if treated seriously and with respect, will enable its readers to understand the true and beautifully complex nature of public health and its associated expertise.

## What is public health?

Public health is the science and art of improving the health of a population. Its expertise is culled from a wide variety of fields of endeavour. It is also a perspective on the world – a way of looking at issues and a way of tackling problems, i.e. thinking about the implications of an individual problem and its solution within the context of the wider population. This is captured in the public health mantra:

- does this issue have implications beyond the immediate?
- does the solution have wider application beyond the immediate?
- is the solution evidence-based and what about evaluation?
- am I the one to address the broader implications and, if so, who else do I need to involve?
- if not, who is?

In addition, those individuals who choose to follow a public health career need to be imbued with a desire to make a positive difference to the human lot. Without this desire, working in the public health field becomes a thankless task. Why so?

Improving the population's health is an extremely complex and difficult task. The health of every individual comprising a defined population is influenced by a variety of determinants. Each of these has numerous dimensions. Figure A illustrates this complexity. A person's health status is the end result of the interaction of genetic make-up, lifestyle and behaviour, together with the physical, psychological, socio-economic, cultural and spiritual components.

In addition to knowledge and skills, effecting positive change within a population requires an inordinate amount of patience, stamina, enthusiasm and energy. Population health is at the mercy of many influences outside the control of individual practitioners. These include government imperatives, resource limitation, lack of the will to change by both the public and other professionals, and individual and organisational vested interests in maintaining the *status quo*. Taking a public health perspective provides an explanation for the often slow nature of change and also removes the focus from self-blame for apparent personal ineffectiveness to make a difference.

The skills and competencies required to practice in a public health way are independent of public policy and organisational frameworks, but to be effective the public health practitioner needs to take account of the context in which they are working.

The long-term focus which epitomises the nature of public health practice is difficult to understand for those working outside the public health field. People know from their own experience what doctors, nurses and other clinicians do. They do not have personal experience of public health and may find it difficult to understand why some health professionals choose to assume the public health mantle and why some choose to leave the clinical field in order to adopt broader responsibilities inherent in public health. There is often a lack of respect for those in public health, vociferously expressed by people working in the clinical field. Public health practitioners are variously viewed as agents of government, pen-pushers, 'drains and sewers' merchants and bureaucrats. They are seen as people who ration resources, who prevent patients from being treated, who quote government circulars and reports and who implement government imperatives. Within this context, it is not an easy decision to choose public health as a career option.

However, there are many notable examples of the success of public health practice. Communicable disease control, maternity and child welfare, school health, food hygiene, healthy eating, smoking cessation, clean air, safe water supplies and health service development are just a few examples of where public health interventions have reduced morbidity and mortality in many populations throughout the world. It is just that the timescales differ so markedly between public health and clinical practice that the outcome has to be measured by different standards.

Public health practice has an established scientific basis but is also an art. A key scientific basis of public health is epidemiology, the study of health and disease in populations. A knowledge of epidemiology enables public health practitioners to measure a population in terms of its health status and to diagnose its sickness levels. It asks the questions '*what* is this sickness?', '*who* has it?', '*where* is it occurring?', '*why* is it occurring?', '*when* is it occurring?' and '*how* is it occurring?' These are not easy questions and they cannot be answered with certainty and accuracy without the application of epidemiological skills and techniques.

However, epidemiology in itself is not capable of providing the full picture. In order to be fully scientifically equipped to make positive change to a population's health, a public health practitioner requires expertise culled from a wide variety of other related fields.

Even if, however, using expertise acquired from all the relevant scientific bases, the answers are forthcoming and the solutions available, it may not be possible to implement action. The art of the public health practitioner is to influence and persuade colleagues, the relevant organisations, politicians and, most importantly, the public that the proposed interventions should be implemented. This requires knowledge and skills distilled from such fields as the behavioural sciences, management and personal development.

The 7P competence model illustrates the diverse and complicated nature of public health practice. It indicates how these myriad areas of expertise are inextricably bound together to create the public health perspective and expertise.

# The 7P model of public health competence

The 7P public health competence model is illustrated in Figure B. What follows is a brief description of each of the seven components of this model.

## Personal development

As has already been noted, taking a public health perspective requires many personal qualities. It is essential to be emotionally mature in order to handle all types of situations effectively. Emotional maturity includes knowing oneself and one's strengths and weaknesses, which enables the development of self-confidence and self-respect. Self-respect is a prerequisite for respecting others. Change happens through people and is dependent on developing good relationships. It is only through working from a basis of respect for self and others that effective relationships can be forged.

Another important area of personal development includes the skill of taking care of oneself. Looking after oneself enables individuals to conserve their energy and to look after others. If you become exhausted, you cannot achieve your goals. Good time management is based on self-respect, self-care and energy management. If you have self-respect, you will look after yourself. You will not overload your diary and you will be able to delegate to others.

You can be a brilliant scientist and discover what needs to be done to solve a problem, but if you cannot communicate this to others so that they have a clear picture of your proposals then you have little hope of achieving change. All those involved in public health need to be articulate both orally and in writing in order to present their work effectively.

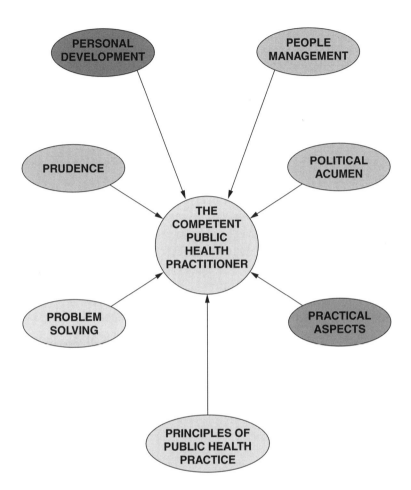

**Figure B:**    The 7P model of public health competence.

## People management

Working effectively with people is not a natural ability. As with all other areas of expertise it has to be learned. This component of the model includes leadership and motivation, managing conflict, working with teams and groups and managing difficult behaviour (*see* Chapter 10).

## Practical aspects

A variety of practical abilities are required for public health competence. These include office management (computer literacy, paper management, managing your personal assistant/secretary, diary management, filing systems, correspondence and telephone management) and financial management (budgets, balance sheets, etc.) – *see* Chapter 10.

## Political acumen

This refers to a variety of issues including understanding the organisation in which you work, knowing who has the power to make things happen and how to gain their support, understanding hidden agendas and vested interests and knowing the right time to take action. This is politics with a small 'p' – the basis of managing change affecting health and healthcare.

## Principles of public health practice

As has already been noted, public health expertise is derived from the integration of knowledge and skills from a wide variety of related fields. Appreciating the relevance of the theory and principles of each of these fields and being able to harness the expertise of others are essential prerequisites for effective public health practice. These fields include clinical medicine, communicable disease control, sociology, psychology, environmental health, nutrition, public health law, health promotion, epidemiology and statistics, ecology, media studies, political theory, public health and social history, research methodology and management theory. As new related fields develop, these will need to be incorporated into the curriculum.

## Problem solving

Problem solving is the basis of public health action. In order to solve a problem it is essential to take a clear and logical approach, breaking down the process into manageable stages. These stages include defining the problem, setting clear and achievable objectives, identifying success criteria, seeking appropriate information, planning for action, implementing action and reviewing the outcome in terms of objectives and success criteria (*see* Chapter 10).

## Prudence

Prudence or wisdom comprises the integration of experience, sensitivity to people, compassion and judgement. A person may have many years of experience and yet may be insensitive to people, without compassion and have faulty judgement. Without prudence, public health will fail in its endeavours.

Each of these seven areas is important in itself but incomplete on its own. Each provides useful pointers for learning for all health professionals but it is essential that all seven areas are integrated to create the whole picture for a 'rounded' public health perspective and effective action. It is the task of a public health training programme to ensure that all areas are covered in its curriculum while at the same time ensuring an integrated approach. The most effective means of achieving this is through problem-based learning.

# Using this book

Modern adult education eschews the traditional passive teaching approach epitomised by standard lectures given by experts to rows of silent students.[2-4] It has been well established that human beings learn best through facilitated self-directed dialogue utilising real experience.[5-9] This book uses real problems to illustrate the knowledge and skills required by public health professionals in their daily work and for all those who need to take a public health perspective. Within the current multidisciplinary context a much wider variety of professions and disciplines have become involved in management, partnership working, and making decisions involving funding and clinical priorities. The examples used here provide a learning framework to help them make best use of these new opportunities for influencing health status at a population level.

There are a variety of ways in which the material provided here can be used. The book can be used for private study and as the basis for interactive seminars and lectures. However, the most effective means of achieving a positive outcome from problem-based learning is through the creation of small peer groups. The individuals in these groups work together to solve problems using the expertise of a facilitator. The group identifies for itself the knowledge and skills required to tackle a given problem and turns to the facilitator for assistance as required. The group, not the facilitator, leads the process. In the traditional teaching mode, the teacher decides the content of the lesson and tells the students what they need to know. A problem-solving approach to learning requires a proactive approach from both the students and the facilitator and background materials must be made available to the students to guide their work. The job of a problem-based learning facilitator is to guide the student through the learning process. If problem-based learning is well managed, it is much more satisfying for both student and teacher and much more fun.

Learning should be an enjoyable process of discovery. It should be hard and exciting work, not a hard and boring grind. The purpose of this book is to take readers on a journey of self-managed discovery.

# The ten areas of public health practice

We have designed this book around the ten areas of public health practice as designated by the English Faculty of Public Health. There is inevitably some overlap between the chapters because, as has already been noted, all aspects of public health work are closely linked. However, for learning purposes, we have separated each of the ten areas as follows:

- surveillance and assessment of the population's health and well-being underpinned by the management, analysis and interpretation of information, knowledge and statistics

- protecting and promoting the population's health and well-being
- developing quality within an evaluative culture that gets evidence into practice and manages risk
- collaborative working for health
- improving healthcare services and addressing inequalities
- policy and strategy development and implementation
- working with and for communities
- strategic leadership for health
- research, development and education
- managing self, people and resources ethically.

## The format of the book

Each chapter outlines an area of practice, describes the learning objectives and provides an illustrative case study (real public health problem). Also included in each chapter are references, bibliographies and/or recommended reading. In addition, depending on the individual author, key issues are identified, learning task examples are given and questions specific to the case study are posed. However, authors have not been asked to provide a definitive and exhaustive dissertation on their particular topic. What is provided is a guide to the knowledge and skills required to address the problems posed within the framework of each of the areas of public health competence defined above. Generally, there is no one right way of tackling or solving public health problems, but each chapter provides hints or pointers to consider when approaching the task. The reader is invited to incorporate new materials, to seek out additional relevant references, to pose other questions and to design innovative tasks to assist the reader in his/her endeavours to absorb the public health perspective.

Public health is an interactive endeavour not a lone adventure. To reflect this, it is recommended that the learning accrued through using this book is seriously reinforced within a small peer-group setting.

The authors wish you, your patients and the populations for which you work a healthy and prosperous future.

## References

1 Documents produced by the Faculty of Public Health Medicine. Refer to website: http://www.fphm.org.uk.

2 World Health Organization (1973) *Continuing Education for Physicians*, WHO Technical Report Series No. 534, 12.

3 David TJ, Dolmans DHJM, Patel L and van der Vleuten CPM (1998) Problem based learning as an alternative to lecture based continuing medical education. *J R Soc Med.* **91**: 626–30.

4 Davis D, Obrien MA, Freemantle N, Wolf FM, Mazmanian P and Taylor-Vaisey A (1999) Impact of formal continuing medical education. Do conferences, workshops, rounds and other

traditional continuing education activities change physician behaviour or health care outcomes? *JAMA.* **282**: 867–74.

5 Foldevi M, Sommansson G and Trell E (1996) Problem-based medical education in general practice and health care quality assurance. *International Journal of Health Care Quality.* **9**(1): 5–14.

6 Bligh J (1995) Problem based learning in medicine: an introduction. *Postgraduate Medical Journal.* **71**: 323–6.

7 Smits PBA, Verbeek JHA and de Buisonje CD (2002) Problem based learning in continuing medical education: a review of controlled evaluation. *BMJ.* **324**: 153–5.

8 Jayawickramarajah PT (1996) Problems for problem based learning: a comparative study of documents. *Medical Education.* **30**: 272–82.

9 Newman P and Peile E (2002) Valuing learners' experience and supporting further growth: educational models to help experienced adult learners in medicine. *BMJ.* **325**: 200–2.

# CHAPTER 1

# Surveillance and assessment of the population's health and well-being

## Paul Fryers

This chapter encompasses managing, analysing and interpreting information, knowledge and statistics, and describes public health surveillance and monitoring, and interpretation of patterns in parameters that reflect the health status of a population. It uses examples from a profile document developed to describe the impact of coronary heart disease on the health of a population to illustrate points about information availability, quality and analysis.

## Learning objectives

- To understand the availability and limitations of routinely collected data and other types of health-related information.
- To understand the analysis and interpretation of data.
- To understand the links between the wider determinants of health, risk factors for disease and health needs.

## Introduction

Ever since John Snow noted the apparent excess in cholera cases in the Golden Square area of London in 1854, the importance of health surveillance has been well documented. His investigation brought together analysis of trends, geographical analysis and qualitative information for a specific need – to identify the source of the infection and define appropriate interventions to stop the spread.[1] In this case the source was the Broad Street pump and the intervention was to disable the pump by removing the handle. This illustrates the essential difference between a public health approach and the case management of individual patients. By the use of statistical, geographical and qualitative information,

John Snow was able to discover the source of the cholera and institute measures to curtail the outbreak. While there is still a need to monitor infectious diseases, similar techniques are now also applied to other factors affecting the health and quality of life of the population, particularly those contributing to high rates of mortality and morbidity.

In this way, current public health professionals, using routinely collected data and other information, are able to identify and measure population-level health needs. Interpreting such information enables the planning of healthcare and other services to improve health and reduce inequalities (*see* Chapter 5). This information is often made available in the form of reports and profiles of communities.

This chapter explores some of the ways in which information is used to describe, monitor and assess the health of the population. For example, an equity profile describes variations or differences in health and risk factors of groups of people within a particular population. This can highlight differences between groups, but further work is then needed to identify the causes of inequalities and interventions by which they may be reduced. It may then be possible to target resources to this end. Examples from a profile for coronary heart disease (CHD) are provided.

The profile was produced as part of Doncaster's CHD strategy. The aim was to describe the impact of CHD on the local population, to examine the patterns of use of services, and by doing so inform a strategy for possible realignment of services and targeting of the necessary resources.

Population health and health services of an area cannot be understood without a broad overview of the characteristics of the population. Demographic and socio-economic factors, such as ethnicity, unemployment, education, deprivation and so on (*see* Section 3), are recognised as having very important effects on health. Conversely, these aspects of community life are themselves affected by the health of individuals and the patterns of health in the population. However, there is often little understanding of what is 'normal' or 'good', in absolute terms, for most population indicators of both health and socio-economic status: they can only be assessed relative to other populations or other times. For example, the people of Doncaster cannot, in any absolute sense, be said to have 'good' health or 'bad' health – we can only say that, in general, they have 'better' health than previous generations, but 'worse' health than people in most other areas of England.

The examples from the CHD Profile form Appendix 1 and are referred to throughout the chapter to illustrate the points discussed.

There are many sources of information available, only a small selection of which are discussed in this chapter. Appendix 2 provides a reference for a broader range of sources of information.

# Section 1: To understand the availability and limitations of routinely collected data and other types of health-related information

This section addresses some of the issues concerning data that might be used to describe the health of a population.

The CHD Profile describes the heart health of the Doncaster population and presents national figures as a comparison. The document was produced using routine data sources (*see* Appendix 2) along with data from previous *ad hoc* projects such as an audit of CHD registers, and a local lifestyle survey – no data were collected specifically for the profile. This pragmatic approach permits a report to be produced relatively quickly, but there are gaps where information is not available.

Most of the examples presented in Appendix 1 make use of data from the Office for National Statistics (ONS). ONS provides routine data across the whole of the UK on a wide range of subjects – for example, population estimates and projections, conceptions and births, deaths, census data, infectious disease notifications, and the results of national surveys such as the General Household Survey.

Other sources of information include hospital activity data, prescribing data, and aggregated data from the Public Health Common Data Set (PHCDS), now incorporated into the *Compendium of Clinical and Health Indicators*.[2] The PHCDS has been a mainstay of public health intelligence since the late 1980s. It includes a massive range of indicators, at health community and local authority level, with rates and confidence intervals ready-calculated. It is usually the first port of call when numbers are needed.

---

Exercise 1.1

- How relevant are the various figures presented from the CHD Profile to the health of the population, and what further information would be useful?

- CHD is an important component of health status in most developed communities, but if the request was for an overall description of the health of the population, what other information would be necessary?

Hints

- Think of the 'healthy' population as well as those with illness.
- Think about the sources of information identified in Appendix 2.
- Consider health-related behaviour, environmental factors and broader determinants of health such as unemployment, deprivation and education (*see* Section 3).
- Consider the historical perspective – for example, the history of coal mining (*see* Section 3).
- Think about data on trends and their part in profiling health in communities (*see* Section 2).

Hospital activity data from the CHD Profile are presented as admission rates (*see* Figures 1.7 and 1.8 in Appendix 1). As well as admissions, there are several other currencies, indicators or units of measurement used in counting NHS activity. These include discharges and deaths, consultant episodes, attendances, contacts and others. The *NHS Data Dictionary and Manual* gives detailed explanations of all these currencies.[3]

In the report, much use is made of death rates, but this simple measure represents only the tip of an iceberg. A refinement, still based solely upon deaths, is 'years of life lost', whereby deaths early in life are weighted more than those in older people. Other methods measure morbidity, including incidence rates for diseases where this can be measured (e.g. cancer, where registers exist throughout the UK, Europe and beyond[4]) and hospital activity rates. There are also measures such as Quality Adjusted Life Years[5] (QALYs), Years Lived with Disability, and Disability Adjusted Life Years[6] (DALYs), which have been used to compare the impact of diseases on different societies. These measures are not intended to allocate different values to different lives, but to try and assess, at a population level, the relative importance of different conditions and the potential benefits from prevention. They can support decision making in resource allocation. Their calculation involves allocating values to different disabilities or conditions, and using these values in conjunction with life expectancy to enable comparison of very different conditions. Hence cataract operations, which do not save lives, but 'improve' life dramatically for many patients, can be discussed in the same terms as smoking cessation campaigns, intensive care facilities or a road bypass.

These measures tend to be used in the context of a disease or a group of diseases, but it is also important to be able to measure health in those who do not overtly have 'a disease'. There are several questionnaires commonly used to ascertain levels of health and general well-being.[7] These include the GHQ (General

Health Questionnaire),[8] EuroQol or EQ5D[9] and the Short Form SF36,[10] which are either freely available or can be commercially obtained. There are no routine data available using these tools at local level, but if setting out to measure levels of general well-being in a local community, it is essential that a validated instrument is used in order for the results to be robust and comprehensible.

In recognition of the importance of social and environmental factors in assessing people's well-being, the concept of 'social capital'* and its measurement is also increasingly being used.

---

**Exercise 1.2**

- Why should public health be interested in 'healthy' people who have not had contact with health services?
- How would you assess the burden on a community of a chronic or disabling disease?

**Hints**

- Think about subclinical and undeclared disease, disability and risk factors.
- Think about the impact on individuals, families, the community and health and social services.

---

The data and information referred to above not only provide a description of the health status of the population, they also allow us to estimate the size of both problems and needs. Prevalence and incidence data are essential for this, supported by the use of routinely collected activity data on the use of services. Appendix 2 gives some details of the availability of incidence and prevalence data.

- *Incidence* is the number of events (e.g. new cases) arising in a given period. Incidence rates are calculated as the number of events in the period divided by the population at risk during that period (and usually multiplied by a constant, such as 100 000, to aid interpretation).
- *Prevalence* is the number of people with a defined condition at a given point in time ('point prevalence'), or who have the condition at some point in a given period ('period prevalence'). Hence (point) prevalence rates are calculated as the number of people with a condition divided by the population at risk (and again usually multiplied by a constant, such as 100 000).

---

* Social capital is a term used to encompass the complex range of factors which contribute to the structure and cohesion of communities, including 'community spirit'. The concept is discussed by Grootaert.[11]

In general, prevalence is most important for chronic conditions where you have a population living with the disease, such as angina. Incidence is more useful for acute episodes, such as acute myocardial infarction (AMI).

---

**Exercise 1.3**

- Consider how quality-of-life measures may be used as part of a health profile of a population. What are the practical difficulties?
- Consider the relationship between prevalence and incidence of a disease and the use of services. For which diseases is there a direct relationship? For which diseases is this less obvious? What are the implications for planning services?

**Hints**

- Consider geographical factors, e.g. remote areas in comparison with those close to hospitals.
- Think about the nature of the disease process and whether a starting point or key event can be identified.

---

# Limitations and pitfalls of use and interpretation of information

Routine data on prevalence of CHD do not exist in most parts of the UK. This represents a major weakness in the epidemiologist's ability to describe the disease in a population. The National Service Framework for CHD set out the requirement for all areas of the country to establish CHD registers, whereby GPs must keep or contribute to an ongoing register of all patients diagnosed with CHD. Figure 1.6 presents data from an audit of these registers conducted immediately after their inception (*see* Appendix 1). At the current stage of the project, we know that there are large variations in completeness of the registers and it is assumed that this is the reason for the variation in rates across practices, once the age distribution of the population has been taken into account. However, there may be other reasons (*see* Exercise 1.4). Melzer *et al.* give a discussion of the opportunities and pitfalls presented by registers, focusing particularly on cancer registries.[4]

When analysing hospital activity data, it is important to bear in mind that coding can be inconsistent between hospitals and from one year to the next. The accuracy of coding may also be affected by changes in coding policy – information on highly political performance indicators can be markedly affected by such changes.

Hospital admission rates for AMI can be used as a proxy for AMI incidence rates, but this misses two groups of people – those who suffer heart attacks so serious that they die without being admitted to hospital, and those with mild attacks which don't result in admission. The rates presented may represent a fair comparison of areas' incidence rates if the proportions dying outright or not being admitted are constant.

Hospitals do collect and provide information on outpatient and accident and emergency department (A&E) attendances, but these are usually less completely coded and tend not to have diagnostic information. Even with fully coded inpatient data, coding practice can vary between hospitals and over time. This should normally be the first area of investigation when dramatic differences between hospitals or between periods are apparent.

Even correctly coded data can be misleading when other factors vary: the NHS performance indicator on delayed discharges following hip replacement originally counted only patients who were discharged home within 56 days from the hospital where the procedure was carried out. A local practice of transferring patients quickly to the community hospital trust for recuperation resulted in these patients not being counted as discharged home within 56 days, until the indicator definition was altered to include discharges home from community hospitals within 56 days of the original procedure. Initially, good practice (and correct coding) resulted in very 'poor performance'.

Most of the examples from the CHD Profile give information for geographically defined populations. Primary care trusts (PCTs) have responsibility for patients registered with their constituent practices, regardless of where they live, so their populations do not usually conform to geographical boundaries. This is a fundamental change in the definition of the population base which public health intelligence and other NHS information will take a little time to come to terms with – not all data sets are easily or accurately attributable to general practices.

The area of health service activity where most patients are seen and treated, and where least information is available, is primary care. The use of information technology in general practices is developing rapidly, and it may be that, in the future, data can be routinely extracted from their computer systems for epidemiological analysis. Until then, the PRIMIS project[12] using the MIQUEST software[13] can be used to extract information from practice systems, and there are projects in many areas to make use of this.

### Exercise 1.4

- Think of other explanations for the variations in CHD prevalence between practices.
- Go through the examples from the CHD Profile. What are the limitations and strengths of the information presented?
- Which of the data sources listed in Appendix 2 can be linked with general practices?
- What problems are likely to arise as a result of the difficulty in providing information on PCTs' registered populations in both urban and rural areas?
- What data should be included in a primary care minimum data set?
- What are the problems with using admission rates as a proxy for prevalence?

### Hints

- Consider the extent to which the examples from the CHD Profile describe the impact of CHD on the population of Doncaster.
- Consider the reasons for inaccurate or unreliable outpatient activity data and how this might be improved.
- Think about sources of prevalence and incidence data.
- Think about data collection and ambiguities in diagnosis or taxonomy.
- Think about the role of audit and incentives.
- Think about GPs' contractual status and incentives.
- Think about the settings in which angina is diagnosed and treated.

# Section 2: To understand the analysis and interpretation of data

This section explains some of the more common methods used for the analysis and interpretation of data. This always has to be done with an eye on the limitations highlighted in the previous section. As examples, maps are presented highlighting wards with 'significantly' higher mortality than the average, and graphs give rates or forecasts which are standardised for age and sex, and presented with confidence intervals where possible. The purposes of and methodologies underlying these are outlined below.

## Mortality rates

As mentioned earlier, many of the examples in Appendix 1 use mortality rates. In its simplest form a mortality rate is a number of deaths (the numerator) in a given time period divided by the population under observation* (the denominator). This, for example, in a population of 1 000 000: if within a year 7500 deaths are observed then the death rate is 7500/1 000 000=0.0075. For ease of understanding, the rates are usually multiplied by a constant factor which, in the case of death rates, is most commonly 100 000. Hence the death rate above would be expressed as 750 deaths per 100 000 population in that year. This is usually referred to as the 'crude death rate'.

Assume that the national death rate is known to have been 300 per 100 000 population for the same period. Our initial observation is that the death rate in our local population is higher. There are many reasons why we might have obtained this result. However, two of these reasons arise so commonly that data analysis is routinely refined to take account of them: the higher death rate could be explained by the age distribution of the population, or it could simply be a result of random variation – a chance finding. The first of these is accounted for by standardising the rates, and the second most commonly by calculating confidence intervals.

---

**Exercise 1.5**

- Why do the rates vary from area to area?

**Hint**

- Think about random variation, risk factor variation, access to and uptake of services, environmental factors, socio-economic factors, etc.

---

* It is critical to have accurate denominator populations. Appendix 2 lists and discusses sources of population data.

# Standardisation

One of the most important factors in explaining death rates is the age–sex distribution of the population. One would clearly expect to see a higher death rate in an area with several nursing homes than in a student area. We account for this in one of two ways. The first is to adjust our local rate by calculating what it would be if our population had the same age–sex distribution as the national (or standard) population. This is called 'direct standardisation' and is the method used throughout the CHD Profile. The results can be expressed as directly standardised rates per 100 000 population, as in the examples given here, or as a 'comparative mortality factor', which gives the death rate relative to a standard rate (100% is the same as the standard rate, 140% means 40% more deaths than in the standard population, 60% means 40% less).

The second method is to use national age-specific death rates to calculate how many deaths we would expect, given the age–sex distribution of our population, and compare that with the number of deaths we actually observed. These are most commonly expressed as standardised mortality ratios (SMRs), for which the interpretation is identical to the comparative mortality factor described above, but can easily be presented as rates per 100 000 population.

The details of calculation of the two methods are covered elsewhere.[14–17] There has been much discussion around the use of the two methods; in recent years direct standardisation has tended to be used more, and indirect standardisation less. There are some particular circumstances when indirect standardisation is computationally easier and, unlike direct standardisation, it can be used if the local age–sex distribution of deaths is not known. However, in general, when comparing many areas, it is more correct and no more difficult to use direct standardisation.

Figure 1.3 presents CHD mortality rates for different areas within Doncaster, standardised for age and sex (*see* Appendix 1).

---

**Exercise 1.6**

- Data are most commonly standardised for age and sex. What other factors might it be useful to standardise for?
- What information is lost by standardising? When would you want to present crude (unstandardised) rates?

---

# Confidence intervals

Many of the charts in Appendix 1 (e.g. Figures 1.3, 1.7 and 1.8) present values for several different areas. Even if the underlying values in each area were the same, we should expect variation in any one time period, purely through randomness, in the same way that if we toss a coin ten times, we would not necessarily get five heads and five tails every time, even though the probability of each outcome is exactly 50%. This kind of random variation occurs in any process that is not completely deterministic, and certainly applies to deaths and most of the other events described here.

A confidence interval has a given probability of containing the 'true' (or 'underlying') value for a population. By convention, the given probability is most commonly 95%, for no particular reason, but it is helpful to have a consistent standard. It does not mean that the population value cannot be outside the range given; purely by chance it will be so 1 in 20 times. If there is a particular desire to be more confident or certain that the range includes the true value, 99% or even 99.9% confidence intervals can easily be constructed.

Hence, when presenting the results of a lifestyle survey, rather than saying that the prevalence of smoking among Doncaster men is 29% (our 'best estimate'), we should emphasise that it is probably between 26% and 32%. The reason for the use of the confidence interval here is clear – the data come from a random sample of the population and we are extrapolating to the whole population. There is commonly a misunderstanding of the need for confidence intervals when there is not obviously a sample being used. For example, when comparing the rate of hospital admissions in one area with that in another, we are using all the admissions and the denominator is the whole population, so why do we need confidence intervals? The answer is straightforward: we know that certain people were hospitalised in that period, but see these as the people who 'happened to be' hospitalised in that period as a result of a more general 'underlying' rate of hospitalisation in that community. They were the cases but, through chance, there could have been more or fewer. Hence we use 95% confidence intervals to give a range within which we believe the general 'underlying' rate falls with 95% probability.*

One key assumption when calculating confidence intervals is that the events are 'independent' – that is, that one event does not *directly* influence the probability of another. There are many instances where this assumption is not valid – for example, death rates from infectious diseases, where an outbreak in one area, with dozens of deaths, does not necessarily imply any underlying tendency for more cases, even though the number of cases may well be 'significantly' higher than anywhere else at that time. When prescribing rates are being compared in

---

* There are other ways of accounting for the random variation in these processes. One which is increasingly coming to the fore is the control chart, which tries to distinguish 'common cause variation' from 'special cause variation'. The terminology and presentation are different but the logic and principles are the same as using confidence intervals. Mohammed *et al.*[18] give a good example of their use.

general practice, 'events' may be prescriptions, tablets or milligrammes of a chemical substance. Obviously these 'events' cannot be considered independent, due to repeat prescriptions or many tablets on one prescription and so on. As there is no way of attributing routine prescribing data to patients or numbers of patients, it is impossible to assess the significance or otherwise of differences in prescribing rates.

# Trends

Figure 1.5 gives an analysis of trend data for mortality (*see* Appendix 1). Data from the past 20 years have been used in order to forecast future rates. There are many ways in which trends can be analysed, as discussed by Chatfield.[19] The most common is through the fitting of a linear regression model on either numbers of cases or rates, or on a log transformation of the rates. If the data appear to fit well to a regression model then the model gives a good assessment of the past trend. However, it is often not the past that is of interest in itself, but only what it can tell us about the future. When forecasting future values it is preferable to use forecasting techniques such as exponential smoothing as has been used here, which can give confidence intervals for the forecasts.

---

**Exercise 1.7**

- Why are the death rates for coronary heart disease falling, as they appear to be from Figure 1.5 (*see* Appendix 1)?

**Hint**

- Think about the relevant importance of behavioural risk factor prevalence (e.g. smoking, diet, exercise), co-morbidities (e.g. diabetes), genetic factors (have levels of susceptibility changed?), environmental factors (socio-economic, pollution, stress), medical and surgical interventions (bypass surgery, thrombolysis, statins), etc.

---

# Geographical data and small-area analysis

The report includes several maps presenting information for different smaller areas within the health community. Although it is easy to display the same information using graphs, the maps are particularly easy to relate to.

Figure 1.9 presents information at electoral ward level (*see* Appendix 1). This is also the level to which ONS Neighbourhood Statistics refer.[20] However, there are often massive variations within wards. For example, the ward of Stainforth, to the North East of Doncaster, has Stainforth itself, a fairly poor and generally deprived community, the largest in the ward, together with several rather more affluent villages. This variation is masked when looking at the ward which appears 'average' on measures of deprivation or health outcomes. Because many of the data are now available at individual level, it is possible to calculate rates for very small areas (e.g. for Stainforth itself as a collection of census enumeration districts). However, areas smaller than wards are seldom useful for analysis, as rates are based on few events and hence have very wide confidence intervals.

Figure 1.4 gives an example of mapping data at small-area level and producing a spatially smoothed 'surface map', showing spatial trends and highlighting pockets of apparently high rates (*see* Appendix 1). It is important to bear in mind that such maps do not give any indication of statistical significance and hence care is necessary when investigating issues identified by them.*

Rather than calculating death rates with huge confidence intervals for small areas, it is preferable to rely on the established links (from large-scale research) between socio-economic deprivation and health (*see* Section 3) and present data from the census (or indicators derived from the census) which are robust at small-area level as in Figure 1.1 (*see* Appendix 1).

---

Exercise 1.8

- What health issues or problems are appropriate for small-area analysis?

---

# Quantitative and qualitative information

The CHD Profile is based on routine information and makes use exclusively of quantitative data. Qualitative and quantitative information have very different roles and the distinction is often not clearly made. The two are complementary and each has its limitations.

In a research context the fundamental difference between qualitative and quantitative information is in the overall aim – whether the researcher is trying to come up with ideas, hypotheses or possible explanations (the role of qualitative research), or to obtain generalisable findings, for example about interventions, populations or relationships between events (the role of quantitative research). There are two unacceptable but common practices: first, the tendency to label poor-quality, non-robust quantitative research as qualitative, in an attempt to

---

* There are geographical information system (GIS) methods available to identify significant clusters of events, which are currently developing rapidly and becoming available to local health intelligence functions.

fend off criticism of statistical design; and, second, giving in to the temptation to report qualitative research findings as generalisable – for example, 'the study shows that patients prefer x type of service to y' rather than 'the study suggests that x type of service might be worth considering over y'.

Outside the research context, quantitative and qualitative information are both needed, treated in appropriate ways. Routine information on hospital outpatient data might show that people in a certain part of a town have high 'did-not-attend' rates. Extensive epidemiological analysis might fail to come up with any reason, whereas qualitative information about bus timetables and reliability might reveal a plausible explanation and possible interventions.

---

**Exercise 1.9**

- How could qualitative information be gathered to try to identify some of the reasons for the differences highlighted in the examples in Appendix 1?
- What are the differences between good qualitative research and good investigative journalism?
- What are the factors which prejudice the generalisability of quantitative information?

**Hint**

- Think particularly about the role of qualitative information in areas that involve public or patients' attitudes or behaviour.

---

# Section 3: To understand the links between the wider determinants of health, risk factors for disease and health needs

Wide use is made in health profiles of data on deprivation, unemployment, ethnicity, etc. (e.g. Figures 1.1 and 1.2 in Appendix 1). These are not traditionally measures of health, but the links between socio-economic factors and health outcomes are well established (*see* Chapter 5). When we know that something, e.g. CHD, is linked strongly with social deprivation, we can assume that need is greatest in areas with the greatest deprivation. As mentioned in Section 2, this is more reliable than trying to analyse CHD mortality rates at a small-area level.

There are many ways of measuring socio-economic status. Income would be a very strong indicator, but we have no information on the income of individuals from their death certificates or hospital records. One of the traditional indicators, the Registrar General's Social Class, is difficult to use because there are no denominator data (i.e. population estimates) between censuses. It is also increasingly limited in its applicability to modern society, and hence is being replaced by the National Statistics Socio-economic Classification.[21] In practice, moreover, most of the data used for analysis have no social class coded. However, most data used for analysis have the individual's postcode, so, rather than analyse individuals' socio-economic status, we can use the level of deprivation found in the small area in which they live. In Figures 1.3, 1.7 and 1.8, small areas have been grouped into five quintiles of deprivation, defined using the Index of Local Deprivation[22] or Townsend Score,[23] such that the people who live in the most deprived areas (wherever in the district they are) are grouped together (*see* Appendix 1). Of course, some wealthy people will be included in the deprived areas and vice versa, but overall the approximation is good enough to demonstrate relationships.

Other examples of indicators of socio-economic status are listed and discussed in Appendix 2.

---

**Exercise 1.10**

- Figure 1.3 shows that CHD mortality rates are markedly higher in deprived groups than in affluent groups of the population. Figure 1.8 does not show the same relationship between revascularisation rates and deprivation, and Figure 1.9 illustrates the absence of a relationship between the two. If the mortality rates indicate levels of need, why might this not be reflected in the revascularisation rates? (*See* Appendix 1.)

- Does finding a relationship between deprivation and CHD mortality rates justify action in deprived communities? If so, what action?

**Hints**

- Think about the confidence intervals and whether this could plausibly be a chance finding.

- Think of other possible explanations – e.g. reasons for differential delays such as less well-educated people ignoring the warning signs of heart attacks; preferential access to services for affluent people; differences in the forms of the disease and hence suitability for revascularisation.

---

The mortality and morbidity measures in the report indicate the burden of CHD on Doncaster's population. They do not suggest ways of trying to reduce the incidence of CHD. Here, as with most diseases, we are dealing with complex causal processes with many factors. The literature can tell us the most important risk factors and we can either use routine information to find groups at particular risk, or survey the population we are interested in.

In the CHD Profile there is information on socio-economic risk factors, as discussed above, but also on individual risk factors such as smoking, exercise and other lifestyle factors, and diabetes. CHD risk is greatly increased in people with diabetes, a condition which is much more common in Asian communities than in other ethnic groups. Hence preventive programmes might appropriately be targeted at such high-risk groups.

Smoking cessation programmes can be targeted at communities where smoking is most prevalent. Although this may not be the most cost-effective way of reducing overall smoking levels and hence CHD incidence, it is the only way in which inequalities can be reduced.

It is very important to understand the population, its history and its possible futures. In Doncaster, the history is of a dominant coal-mining industry, with certain specific conditions linked to the type of work (e.g. pneumoconiosis and chronic obstructive pulmonary disease (COPD)) but confounded with smoking. More recently, the closure of coal mines has resulted in localised mass long-term unemployment and consequent health effects.*

Finally, it is likely that genetic risk factors will become better understood in the future, and screening programmes will be able to identify those at high risk of a wide range of diseases.

---

**Exercise 1.11**

- How can different agencies work together to improve health through knowledge and understanding of socio-economic factors such as education attainment levels, housing conditions and unemployment, together with health outcomes information?
- How would you present the case for overall population reduction of smoking, and the case for targeted reduction in high-prevalence groups, to reduce this risk factor for CHD?
- What are the potential positive and negative implications of genetic screening programmes?

---

In terms of employment, any new developments are to be welcomed as they may be expected to generate investment and regeneration. However, they may also bring new environmental hazards (e.g. pollutants, risk of accidents, increased traffic). Estimating the balance between these benefits and disbenefits is based on the results of environmental and health impact assessments (*see* Chapters 5 and 6).

Health impact assessment is emerging as an increasingly important area of public health work. In the UK there is no legal requirement to have a health impact statement for, say, an industrial development, even though it is required to have an environmental impact statement. However, it is rapidly becoming a major area of public health practice, as planning committees increasingly request health impact statements. Methods are evolving quickly – the British Medical Association (BMA) has published a useful guide and Abdel Aziz *et al.* give a practical example.[25,26] In many cases, background information about the health of the population will be required in a very similar format to the examples in Appendix 1.

---

* In the Dearne Valley area between Barnsley, Doncaster and Rotherham, for example, in 1981, over 8000 men worked in the coal-mining industry, some 25% of the total workforce. By 1991, when the last pit in the area closed, 93% of these jobs had gone and by 1997 there were around 50 men left working in the industry.[24]

Exercise 1.12

- There is a proposal to develop a major airport in the South East ward of Doncaster. Write a project proposal indicating the data you would require, and what methods may be used to obtain them, in order to describe aspects of the development which might have an impact on coronary heart disease.

Hints

- Which of the examples in Appendix 1 are useful?
- If it is expected that the airport will cause an increase in morbidity – e.g. CHD rates – is it appropriate to consider the existing rates of CHD in the locality? Is it any more acceptable to risk negative health impacts in an area with 'good health' than in one with already 'poor health'?
- Refer to other chapters in this book, particularly Chapters 4, 5, 6, 7 and 9.

# References

1 Snow J (1855) *On the Mode of Communication of Cholera* (2e). John Churchill, London.

2 Lakhani A and Olearnik H (eds) (2002) *Compendium of Clinical and Health Indicators 2001*. Department of Health, London.

3 NHS Information Authority (2002) *The NHS Data Dictionary and Manual Version 1.3*. NHS Information Authority, Birmingham. http://www.nhsia.nhs.uk/datastandards/pages/ddm/index.htm.

4 Melzer D, Newton J and Davies T (2001) Assessing longer-term health trends: registers. In: D Pencheon, CS Guest, D Melzer and JAM Gray (eds) *Oxford Handbook of Public Health Practice*. Oxford University Press, Oxford.

5 Phillips C and Thompson G (2001) What is a QALY? *Evidence-based Medicine*. **1**(6). http://www.evidence-based-medicine.co.uk/ebmfiles/WhatisaQALY.pdf.

6 Murray CJL and Lopez AD (1996) *The Global Burden of Disease: a comprehensive assessment of mortality and disability from diseases, injuries and risk factors in 1990 and projected to 2020*. Harvard School of Public Health on behalf of the World Health Organization and the World Bank, Cambridge, MA.

7 Donald A (2001) What is quality of life? *Evidence-based Medicine*. **1**(9). http://www.evidence-based-medicine.co.uk/ebmfiles/WhatisQoL.pdf.

8 Goldberg D and Williams PA (1988) *User's Guide to the General Health Questionnaire*. nferNelson, Windsor. http://www.nfer-nelson.co.uk/ghq/.

9 EuroQol Group (1996) *5D User Guide*. EuroQol, Rotterdam. http://www.euroqol.org/.

10  Ware J, Snow KK, Kosinski M and Gandek B (1993) *SF-36 Health Survey: manual and interpretation guide.* The Health Institute, New England Medical Center, Boston, MA. http://www.qualitymetric.com/marketplace/detail.cgi?pid=SF-002.

11  Grootaert C (1998) *Social Capital: the missing link?* World Bank, Washington, DC. http://www.worldbank.org/poverty/scapital/wkrppr/sciwp3.pdf.

12  PRIMIS. http://www.primis.nottingham.ac.uk/.

13  NHS Information Authority. http://www.nhsia.nhs.uk/nhais/pages/products/vaprod/miquest/.

14  Armitage P and Berry G (1994) *Statistical Methods in Medical Research* (3e). Blackwell, Oxford.

15  Breslow NE and Day NE (1987) *Statistical Methods in Cancer Research; Vol II – the design and analysis of cohort studies* (IARC Scientific Publications 82). International Agency for Research on Cancer, Lyon.

16  Altman DG (1991) *Practical Statistics for Medical Research.* Chapman and Hall, London.

17  Bland M (2000) *An Introduction to Medical Statistics* (3e). Oxford University Press, Oxford.

18  Mohammed MA, Cheng KK, Rouse A and Marshall T (2001) Bristol, Shipman, and clinical governance: Shewhart's forgotten lessons. *Lancet.* **357**(9254): 463–7.

19  Chatfield C (1996) *The Analysis of Time Series: an introduction* (5e). Chapman & Hall, London.

20  National Statistics. http://www.statistics.gov.uk/neighbourhood/home.asp.

21  National Statistics. http://www.statistics.gov.uk/nsbase/methods_quality/ns_sec/default.asp.

22  DETR (1998) *Index of Local Deprivation.* Department of the Environment, Transport and the Regions, London.

23  Townsend P, Phillimore P and Beattie A (1988) *Health and Deprivation: inequality and the North.* Routledge, London.

24  DETR. *Regeneration of Former Coalfield Areas: interim evaluation. Case Study notes: Dearne.* The Stationery Office, London. http://www.urban.odpm.gov.uk/programmes/coalfields/dearne/01.htm (accessed 13 November 2002).

25  BMA (1998) *Health and Environmental Impact Assessment: an integrated approach.* Earthscan, London.

26  Abdel Aziz MI, Radford J and McCabe J (2000) *Health Impact Assessment, Finningley Airport.* Doncaster Health Authority, Doncaster. http://www.doncasterhealth.co.uk/documents/finningley/finningley_report.html (accessed 11 July 2002).

NB: Except where stated, all website addresses quoted were accessed on 24 June 2002.

# Further reading

- Department of Health (2001) *Shifting the Balance of Power.* DoH, London.
- Donaldson LJ and Donaldson RJ (2000) *Essential Public Health* (2e). LibraPharm Limited, Newbury. (Chapter 1: Assessing the health of the population.)
- Longley PA, Goodchild MF, Maguire DJ and Rhind DW (2000) *Geographic Information Systems and Science.* John Wiley, Chichester.

- Pencheon D, Guest CS, Melzer D and Gray JAM (eds) (2001) *Oxford Handbook of Public Health Practice*. Oxford University Press, Oxford. (Particularly Part 1: Public health assessment.)
- Pope C, Ziebland S and Mays N (2000) Qualitative research in health care: analysing qualitative data. *BMJ*. **320**: 114–16.
- Wright J (ed) (1998) *Health Needs Assessment in Practice*. BMJ Books, London.
- Wright J (2001) Assessing health needs. In: D Pencheon, CS Guest, D Melzer and JAM Gray (eds) *Oxford Handbook of Public Health Practice*. Oxford University Press, Oxford.
- See also the references to the wider determinants of health in Chapter 5.

## Acknowledgements

I am grateful to John Cornell and my father Tom Fryers for their help with this chapter. I am also grateful to my colleagues in Doncaster, particularly Heather McCabe and Chris McManus, who provided most of the data used in the examples.

# Appendix 1: Examples from a coronary heart disease profile of Doncaster

## Socio-economic background

CHD risk is influenced by poverty. Using the Index of Local Deprivation, the enumeration districts* (EDs) in Doncaster have been ranked and the most deprived 20% of EDs are shown in Figure 1.1. These areas might be taken as target areas for action.

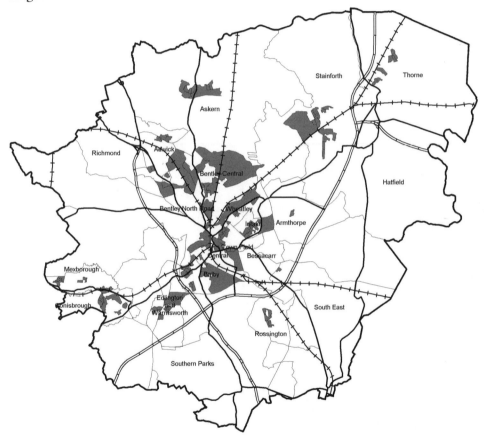

**Figure 1.1:** Doncaster wards with the 20% most deprived census enumeration districts shaded (defined using the DETR Index of Local Deprivation).

* Census enumeration districts are the smallest areas for which 1991 census data can be provided. They average around 400 to 500 population and were designed as convenient areas for census enumerators (the people who collected the forms) to cover. The 2001 census data will be provided in similarly sized output areas, but they will be defined from the data in order to provide demographically more coherent areas.

People's risk of developing CHD also varies with their ethnicity. For example, CHD death rates are about 25% to 50% lower among people of Afro-Caribbean descent than among UK whites. By contrast, some groups of people of South Asian origin have a CHD risk that is about 40% greater than whites in the UK. Figure 1.2 shows the EDs with the majority of ethnic minority communities at the time of the 1991 census.

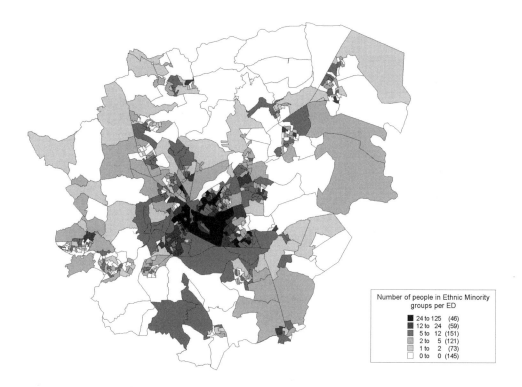

**Figure 1.2:**   The number of people in ethnic minority groups for the enumeration districts in Doncaster, 1991.

# Variations in CHD mortality rates

Figure 1.3 shows how mortality rates from CHD vary within the local authority (LA) borough of Doncaster. Rates have been calculated using direct standardisation and 95% confidence intervals applied. The fact that the entire confidence interval for the Doncaster CHD mortality rate is well above the England and Wales rate indicates that the Doncaster rate is *significantly* higher than the national rate. However, the overlapping confidence intervals for the three PCTs

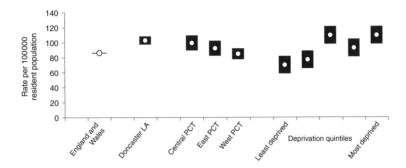

**Figure 1.3:** Mortality rates for coronary heart disease (International Classification of Diseases-9 410–414), 1996–98. All persons aged under 75. Directly standardised rates with 95% confidence intervals.

suggest that there is no significant difference in rates between the three. The enumeration districts in Doncaster have been ranked according to the Townsend Index of deprivation and grouped into quintiles such that quintile 1 includes the most affluent 20% of EDs and quintile 5 the most deprived 20% of EDs. Calculating the mortality rates for the different quintiles of deprivation demonstrates that CHD mortality rates are considerably higher among those who live in deprived areas.

Figure 1.4 shows how data at small-area level can be used to generate a 'surface map'. The tinted contours allow areas with high rates to be identified, when this type of map is used together with maps showing topographic data such as that included on Figure 1.1.*

## Trends

Figure 1.5 shows how the death rates from CHD have fallen over the last 20 years. Line ① gives the rate for the most deprived quintile of EDs (see definition for Figure 1.3) with line ② giving the rate for the other four quintiles combined. Although the deprived group has higher mortality rates throughout the period of analysis, there is some evidence here that the gap might have narrowed very slightly. However, the trends could be affected by changing demographics before

---

* There are more examples like this, along with more explanation, in the South Yorkshire Health Inequalities Atlas, available on http://www.doncasterhealth.co.uk/syhlthineqatlas/index.html (accessed 11 July 2002).

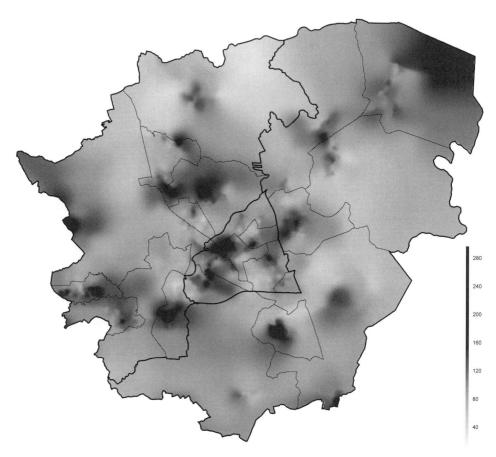

**Figure 1.4:** Mortality rates for coronary heart disease (ICD-9 410–414), 1996–2000. All persons aged under 75. Spatially smoothed, directly standardised rates.

and after the 1991 census.* Lines ③–⑤ show forecasts with 95% confidence intervals to the year 2010.

# CHD in primary care

The National Service Framework for coronary heart disease requires that 'a systematically developed and maintained practice-based CHD register is in place and actively used to provide structured care to people with established CHD by April 2001'. An audit of Doncaster GP practices carried out by the Doncaster

---

* There are more examples like this in the Joint Report of the Directors of Public Health for Barnsley, Doncaster and Rotherham, March 2001, available on http://www.doncasterhealth. co.uk/documents/dph/dph01/jphar.htm (accessed 8 July 2002).

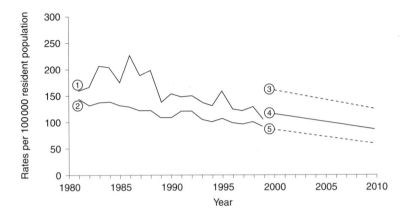

**Figure 1.5:** Mortality rates for coronary heart disease (ICD-9 410–414), 1981–99. All persons aged under 75. Directly standardised rates. Rates for 2000–10 forecast with 95% confidence intervals by Holt's Method on logit-transformed data.

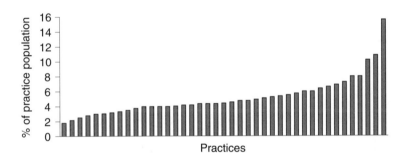

**Figure 1.6:** Percentage of practice lists on the CHD register, 2001. Doncaster general practices.

Medical Audit Advisory Group brought together information on how many patients were included on the registers. The intention is that these lists will include all patients with diagnosed coronary heart disease and may be used to estimate prevalence.

## Hospital activity

In the absence of accurate incidence or prevalence data for CHD, hospital activity data can shed some light on patterns of the disease, as many people suffering heart attacks or angina are admitted to hospital. Figure 1.7 shows that admission rates for coronary heart disease are significantly lower in Central PCT and significantly higher in East PCT than the Doncaster rate. The quintile figures suggest that admission rates for coronary heart disease increase with increasing levels of deprivation, in a similar way to the mortality rates in Figure 1.3.

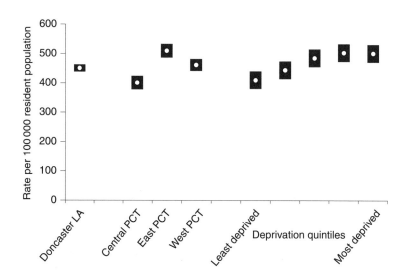

**Figure 1.7:** Admission rates for coronary heart disease (ICD-10 120–125), April 1997 to March 2000. All persons, all ages. Directly standardised rates with 95% confidence intervals.

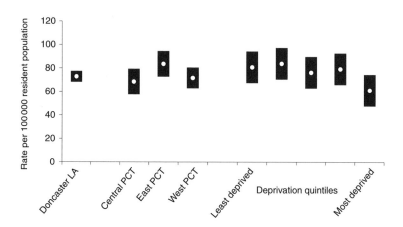

**Figure 1.8:** Admission rates for coronary angioplasty (OPCS-4 K40–K44, K49), April 1997 to March 2000. All persons, all ages. Directly standardised rates with 95% confidence intervals.

Surgical treatment for coronary heart disease is mainly through revascularisation – coronary artery bypass graft (CABG) or percutaneous transluminal coronary angioplasty (PTCA). Admission rates for revascularisation are shown in Figure 1.8, and do not show the same relationship with deprivation as appears in Figures 1.3 and 1.7. In fact there is a decreasing trend with increasing deprivation.

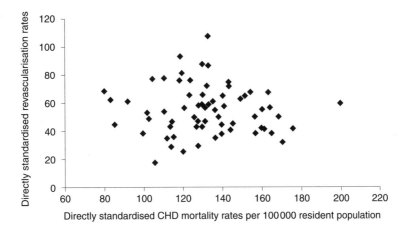

**Figure 1.9:**   Relationship between CHD mortality rates 1992–96 and revascularisation rates 1995–96 to 1997–98. Wards in Barnsley, Doncaster and Rotherham.

Figure 1.9 shows electoral-ward-level revascularisation rates plotted against CHD mortality rates for all wards in the South Yorkshire Coalfields Health Action Zone (Barnsley, Doncaster and Rotherham local authorities). There is no obvious relationship between these two indicators, when one might be expected.

# Appendix 2: Information sources

*Note*: Many of the data described below are described as being available at health authority level or held by health authorities. Following the publication of *Shifting the Balance of Power* (the 2002 reorganisation of health authorities and PCTs) the basis for providing information will be altered, variously, to PCTs, local authorities and/or new (strategic) health authorities. These possibilities must be taken into account by the reader when trying to track down information discussed here as, in most cases, it is not clear at the time of writing what information will be provided at what level, and indeed it may vary in different parts of England.

## Population and demography

| | |
|---|---|
| Census | Data from the 1991 census give populations by age group, sex, social class, ethnic origin, etc., at national, regional, district (health and local authority), electoral ward and enumeration district levels. Data from the 2001 census will become available in late 2002 and 2003 – until then the data are very out of date. |
| Office for National Statistics | ONS issue annual mid-year estimates of population by age group and sex at local and health authority level.   In 1998 they issued estimates of ward populations in three broad age bands.   ONS periodically issue population projections at local and health authority level. |
| Health authority patient registers | Health authorities hold registers of all residents of their catchment area registered with a GP, from which counts by age, sex, geographical area (PCT, ward, enumeration district, postcode) and general practice can be obtained. Patient registers do not include residents not registered with a GP, but still tend to overcount population (partly because of delays in removal from lists), and hence can not be totally relied upon. |
| Local estimates | Health authorities may produce their own estimates by combining the above sources. In addition, some local authorities produce estimates of population based on the electoral register. In some cases, estimates may be produced collaboratively combining all the available information. |

# Mortality

Office for National Statistics

Annual extracts give final death records for all deaths occurring in, or registered in, each calendar year. The individual records can be aggregated by age, sex, cause(s) of death, area of residence, etc. Registered GP name is not included on the death certificate: if it were, analysis of mortality rates by practice or PCT would be more practicable.

The Public Health Mortality File consists of individual death certificate records supplied to health authorities (and from them to PCTs subject to local arrangements) on a monthly basis to support public health surveillance. Causes of death given are not always final; hence the annual extracts are more reliable when they become available.

Summary statistics are provided in various reports, e.g. the vital statistics (VS1, 2, 3, 5) reports, which give counts of deaths by cause and, particularly, summaries of perinatal and infant mortality rates at health authority level.

*Compendium of Clinical and Health Indicators*

The compendium is an annual data set issued to PCTs and local health communities on CD-ROM, consisting of spreadsheets giving counts and rates for a wide range of health indicators for all local health communities and local authorities in England. It includes analyses of deaths for a wide selection of causes, giving age-specific rates, SMRs, directly standardised rates, all with 95% confidence intervals, and years of life lost.

PCT/local health community arrangements for managing patient registrations

Deaths can be identified from the 'deletions' file of patients removed from GPs' lists.

Local register offices

Historically public health surveillance has made use of a regular supply of death certificate records direct from local register offices. This source has largely been rendered superfluous by the Public Health Mortality File, which includes data for residents of the health authority (HA), wherever their death was registered, and includes ICD-coded causes of death.

Confidential enquiry reports

Annual reports from confidential enquiries include data on infant and perinatal deaths, maternal deaths and others.

# Incidence and prevalence

Cancer registries
: Data on all cancer registrations are held by regional cancer registries and can be made available to health authorities. Individual records can be aggregated by age, sex, area of residence, etc., to give good estimates of incidence rates.

Disease registers
: Registers of patients with specific conditions are kept locally, but with no consistency across the country. These include people with diabetes, those with psychiatric illness, abused children, etc. Following the National Service Framework for coronary heart disease, primary-care-based CHD registers are being established where they did not exist previously. They will be unreliable in the short term, but in the longer term registers like this give a good opportunity to monitor incidence and prevalence of a range of important conditions.

Primary care
: In some areas, where GPs have advanced information systems, analysis can be carried out (possibly using analysis tools such as MIQUEST) to estimate the prevalence of certain diseases and conditions. As primary care information systems improve and are used more effectively, there is potential for information on incidence and prevalence of a wide variety of conditions to be made available. Many conditions are primarily treated in general practices and knowledge of them could contribute a great deal to epidemiological understanding of health and illness in society.

Hospital activity
: Health authorities have records of inpatient admissions and outpatient and A&E attendances involving their residents, supplied by acute hospitals. For some acute events that almost universally result in hospitalisation (for example, fractured neck of femur), they may be used to estimate incidence rates, but for most they can only be taken as a poor indicator of need.

Infectious disease notifications
: Details of all cases of notifiable diseases are collected by the local authority or health authority and are usually kept by consultants in communicable disease control (CCDCs).

National surveys
: The General Household Survey gives data at regional level on the prevalence of long-standing and acute illnesses and the extent to which they limit daily activity.

The Health Survey for England collects information on specific disease areas, covering different areas each year. Data are provided at health authority level, but the sample size is extremely small and hence confidence intervals very wide.

ONS also do a range of intermittent national surveys – for example, the psychiatric surveys giving estimates of prevalence for psychiatric disorders.

Local surveys

*Ad hoc* surveys, such as the Sheffield Health and Illness Prevalence Survey (SHAIPS), can give estimates of disease prevalence.

In most areas regular surveys of children's dental health give estimates of prevalence of tooth decay (DMFT scores), kept by dental public health directors.

*Compendium of Clinical and Health Indicators*

The compendium is an annual data set issued to HAs on CD-ROM, consisting of spreadsheets giving counts and rates for a wide range of health indicators for all HAs and LAs in England. It includes some data on incidence, e.g. cancers, fractured neck of femur, meningitis, etc.

Census

The 1991 and 2001 censuses included a question on long-term illness and the extent to which it limits daily activity. Data for 2001 will be made available by mid-2003.

Literature

For many areas of health, the best hope of estimating local incidence or prevalence is from published literature, particularly reviews. Health organisations' library and information services may be able to help.

## Births, conceptions and abortions

Office for National Statistics

Annual extracts give birth records for all births occurring in each calendar year. The individual records can be aggregated by outcome (live or stillbirth), sex, birth weight, area of residence, etc.

The Public Health Birth File gives data from the birth registrations monthly. This is not purchased in many health authorities.

Summary reports, such as VS1 and VS2, give aggregated data on birth weight, maternal age and outcome.

Counts of conceptions (abortions and maternities) are provided by ONS to health authorities at HA and ward level, broken down by maternal age to allow monitoring of teenage pregnancy rates (under 16, under 18 and under 20). At ward level, data are not always made available for confidentiality reasons.

ONS can provide *ad hoc* aggregated analyses on request – for example, aggregated over a longer time period to avoid small number confidentiality problems.

Hospital activity

Inpatient records supplied by hospitals give details of births in hospital.

Population trends

The Spring issues of the journal *Population Trends* have included analysis each year of teenage pregnancy rates for all health authorities in England.

*Compendium of Clinical and Health Indicators*

The compendium is an annual data set issued to HAs on CD-ROM, consisting of spreadsheets giving counts and rates for a wide range of health indicators for all HAs and LAs in England. It includes counts and rates of conceptions, births and abortions.

# Lifestyle and risk factors

National surveys

The General Household Survey gives estimates of smoking and alcohol consumption, at regional level.

The Health Survey for England collects data on risk factors through physical measurements (height, weight, blood pressure, etc.) and a blood sample (cholesterol, serum cotinine for smoking, etc.) in addition to a questionnaire. Data are provided at health authority level, but the sample size is extremely small and hence confidence intervals very wide.

Local surveys

Lifestyle surveys are frequently carried out by health authorities to obtain estimates of lifestyle factors related to health, such as smoking, diet, alcohol, exercise, stress, etc. The expense of obtaining samples large enough to estimate the prevalence of these factors for small areas within health authorities (e.g. wards) is normally prohibitive.

Primary care

In some areas, where GPs have advanced information systems, analysis can be carried out (possibly using analysis tools such as MIQUEST) to estimate prevalence of certain risk factors. As primary care information systems improve and are used more effectively, there is potential for information on incidence and prevalence of a wide variety of conditions to be made available. It must be borne in mind that reporting of health-related behaviour to GPs is not necessarily accurate.

Literature

For many risk factors, the best hope of estimating local incidence or prevalence is from published literature. Health authority library and information services may be able to help.

# Wider determinants of health

Deprivation indices

There are several commonly used deprivation indices based on census data. They include the Townsend and Carstairs indices, developed by researchers in the health field, and the Index of Local Conditions and Index of Local Deprivation, developed for use in local government. Each uses a slightly different combination of census variables, and there is broad agreement between them in their categorisation of local and health authorities, wards and enumeration districts. They are all readily available within health and local authorities or on the Internet.

Other deprivation indicators have been developed for resource allocation, and are probably best used for this purpose – for example, the Jarman Score and the Relative Needs Index.

The Indices of Multiple Deprivation 2000 were developed to overcome the problem of using out-of-date census data, and use 1998 data. They are available at local authority and ward level from local authorities or from ONS Neighbourhood Statistics (http://www.statistics.gov.uk/neighbourhood).

Unemployment

Unemployment rates are very good indicators of general deprivation levels and are available monthly from local authorities. The Nomis system from which the data are taken is intended to be made available through the ONS Neighbourhood Statistics website in the future. Data are available at local authority and ward level.

Census data give unemployment at national, local and health authority, ward and enumeration district level. Data for 2001 will be available by mid-2003.

Education

Educational attainment data (GCSEs, Key Stage 2 scores, absences and exclusions) are available from local authority education departments. These give details of performance of students each year.

Adult numeracy and literacy data can be obtained from the Basic Skills Agency (http://www.basic-skills.co.uk).

Census data give educational attainment levels of people of all ages at national, local and health authority, ward and enumeration district level.

Environment
Local authority environmental services departments collect data on pollution levels (e.g. particulates), usually in only a few locations (e.g. close to busy roads or junctions).

Housing
The census gives details of housing type, size and tenure.

Local authority housing departments have data from housing needs surveys on various aspects of housing, homelessness and distance from work.

Benefits
The Benefits Agency has data on housing benefit and income support, giving an indication of levels of wealth.

Crime
Local authorities commission crime audits which can usually give crime rates by ward. However, crime rates are difficult to interpret, as the appropriate denominator is often not easily defined – for example, car crime is related to where cars are left (shopping, workplace, etc.) rather than only the number of residents or households.

Police information systems hold detailed data on crimes but are often not easily interrogated to give aggregated data at, say, ward level. However, information may be made available to assist enquiries in a particular locality.

Others
The list above is far from comprehensive – there are many more aspects to describing the socio-economic make-up of society. The principal source of data on populations is the decennial census, which gives detailed, small-area data on the above areas and others such as car ownership and single-parent families.

There are also several national surveys, which give annual data, such as the Labour Force Survey which also includes income data.

The ONS Neighbourhood Statistics website (http://www.statistics.gov.uk/neighbourhood) includes a constantly expanding range of data at ward level.

# Health services

Hospital inpatients
Health authorities hold data on all inpatient stays of their residents, received (via a national clearing service) from hospitals. The data are at individual level and may

be aggregated by age, sex, area of residence (e.g. ward, enumeration district, postcode), diagnoses, procedures undertaken, and a great many more variables. The data are reasonably complete and normally taken to be fairly accurately coded, although this will vary from hospital to hospital. These data can be used to compare rates of service utilisation, to identify differences in need for, access to, referral to or provision of services.

Hospital outpatients  Similarly to the inpatient data, health authorities have records of all outpatient attendances of their residents. Although the data can be used in similar ways to the inpatient data, they are less complete and less well coded. Diagnostic coding, for example, is often incomplete.

Accident and Emergency  A&E data sets are, where available at all, limited in the extent to which they are coded, but comparisons of rates of A&E attendance by GP practice can be made in some areas.

Waiting lists  Details are also received by health authorities from hospitals of patients waiting for inpatient admission, including the waiting time, and counts of those waiting for outpatient appointments.

Community and mental health services  Details of contacts are available in some areas to varying standards.

Körner returns  Since the 1980s, these aggregated returns have been used to record health service activity. They cover the above areas of hospital and community activity and other aspects of health service provision.

NHS performance indicators  These indicators, issued annually, but with varying content and timescales, present comparative analyses of health services around the country. They have previously been labelled high-level performance indicators, clinical effectiveness indicators and clinical indicators. They are published by the Department of Health and often receive press interest and coverage. The indicators cover a wide range of service areas, including re-admission rates, post-operative mortality rates, delayed discharges, rates of various complications and many more. Their political weight can be useful in generating interest in variations at a high level within health organisations. The indicators are made available to health authorities directly and some are included in the *Compendium of Clinical and Health Indicators*.

| | |
|---|---|
| Primary care prescribing | Data are available through the national databases (ePACT and ePACT.net) on all prescriptions issued by general practitioners in the PCT area (PACT = Prescribing Analysis and CosT). The data include complete details of the drugs prescribed (number and size of tablets or other units as appropriate) and can be related to age–sex-adjusted populations (patient units – PUs – etc.) to give rates. However, there are no details of the patient involved or the diagnosis, and it is hence not possible to estimate the number of patients being prescribed with any given drug, except in cases where drugs are prescribed only for one purpose and in standard doses. |
| Vaccination and immunisation | Data can be extracted from health authority patient register systems on uptake rates for childhood vaccination and immunisation. |
| Screening | Data on cervical screening uptake rates can be extracted from health authority patient register systems. Aggregated information on attendance rates is available annually on the Körner return, KC61. |
| | Data on breast screening uptake rates are available from the annual KC63 return. |
| Dental registrations | Routine data normally held by district dental advisers or dental public health directors give data on the proportion of adults registered with a dentist. |
| Primary care activity | In some areas, where GPs have advanced information systems, analysis can be carried out (possibly using analysis tools such as MIQUEST) of consultations by diagnosis and treatments. As primary care information systems improve and are used more effectively, there is potential for more information on primary care activity to be made available. Linking primary care consultation data to secondary, tertiary and community service records would allow complete pathways of care to be studied and give opportunities for improving communication between sectors and streamlining systems. |
| Social services | The mutual dependence of health and social services means that apparently poor performance in one sector can be due to failures in the other. Social services performance indicators give a range of comparative indicators for social services departments across the country. Locally, 'Quality Protects' plans give summary data. |

CHAPTER 2

# Promoting and protecting the health of the population

*Rosy McNaught*

## Introduction

Promoting and protecting the health of the population encompasses a wide range of activities, many of which overlap. This chapter focuses on the health protection function. Health protection is an important element of the public health function and has been defined as:

> 'the application of a set of multidisciplinary public health knowledge and skills that aims to protect the public's health from biological, chemical and physical hazards in the environment.'*

This encompasses the control of communicable disease, the health consequences arising from exposure to non-communicable environmental hazards, and the health emergency planning response.

In this chapter, a communicable disease incident is used as a case study, but identical skills are required to respond to a chemical incident or environmental hazard. The principles which underlie the planning of the health emergency response to a major incident allow the development of a flexible plan applicable to dealing with any sort of emergency, whether communicable disease or chemical hazard.

## Learning objectives

By working through the contents of this chapter, the reader should:

- gain an understanding of the role of the health service as part of a multi-agency approach
- understand the issues involved in working across different organisations
- understand the importance of networks as a means of dealing with complex issues

* Public Health Medicine Environmental Group, July 2001.

- gain an understanding of the pivotal role of communications in the health protection function
- gain an insight into the practical problems that are faced and how to approach them
- gain an ability to deal with the emergency/'on-call' situation, responding appropriately and acting in a timely manner
- gain knowledge of local information networks and communication channels
- gain an ability to respond in an outbreak situation, liaising and communicating with other professionals and other agencies and supporting/undertaking timely control measures.

---

**Case study**

**Case A**

Monday 4 January

A 15-year-old boy was admitted to hospital with a fever, vomiting, headache, stiff neck and photophobia. There was no evidence of a rash, and a clinical diagnosis of meningitis was made. He had suffered a flu-like illness over the Christmas weekend, from which he appeared to recover, but on Saturday 2 January, he had been taken ill again. The consultant paediatrician considered that, in view of the history of the preceding viral illness, this was more likely to be viral or pneumococcal infection, rather than the more common meningococcal meningitis.

**Q How would you get to know about this case? Who would notify the 'appropriate person'\* to deal with the situation? How? When would you expect to find out about the case?**

Acute meningitis and meningococcal septicaemia are diseases which are required to be notified to the 'Proper Officer'† of the local authority, under the provisions of the Public Health (Control of Disease) Act 1984 and the Public Health (Infectious Diseases) Regulations 1988.

   This means that the doctor who suspects that a patient is suffering from meningitis is required to submit a written certificate to the local authority, containing details of the patient. However, although this information will eventually filter through to the 'appropriate person', the information will be too late to allow effective action to take place.

\* *The appropriate person to deal with the situation* – this used to be the local department of public health situated in the health authority, but following the NHS reorganisation will depend on local arrangements. This may include the local office of the Health Protection Agency, a primary care trust (PCT) department of public health or Director of Public Health and so on. It is essential that robust arrangements are in place to ensure that everyone who may need to inform the 'appropriate person' knows how to do so (*see* Further Reading – *Getting Ahead of the Curve*).

† The Proper Officer is appointed by the local authority to act on its behalf in protecting the health of the public and in discharging the legal aspects pertaining to the public health. This is usually the local Consultant in Communicable Disease Control (CCDC) and the Director of Public Health.

In practice, the hospital doctor who makes the diagnosis should telephone the public health doctor on call as soon as possible, with the personal and clinical details of the case. There should be arrangements in place for a 24-hour 'on-call' service for public health emergencies, and the hospital doctors should be made aware that telephone notifications of meningitis can be made at any time. Local arrangements may be in place such that public health doctors are not telephoned about cases between, say, midnight and 8 a.m.,[‡] but if so, the details of the case should be telephoned to the department first thing in the morning. During 'daylight' hours, the public health doctor should reasonably expect to be notified by telephone of a case within eight hours of admission.

Occasionally, the public health doctor will become aware of a case by other, 'unofficial' routes. The parents may telephone the school, and the first notification of the case may come from the head teacher, requesting information and advice. Friends and family members, or work colleagues who have been informed of the case, may also act as the primary source of information. In this situation great care must be taken to verify the information given with the hospital staff, and to maintain the confidentiality of the index case.

**Q What investigations would you expect the hospital to carry out to confirm the diagnosis? What are their limitations? When would you expect to get confirmation of the diagnosis? What difference would this make to your actions?**

A number of investigations were carried out, including a blood culture, a polymerase chain reaction (PCR) test looking for meningococcal DNA, meningococcal serology, C-reactive protein (CRP) and virological studies. A lumbar puncture was attempted but was unsuccessful. A throat swab was not taken. The patient was treated with a full course of intravenous antibiotics and he made a full recovery.

**Q Apart from basic clinical details, what specific information would you expect to be given in order to determine the appropriate public health response? What would you do?**

As pneumococcal disease was considered the most likely diagnosis, the department of public health was not informed until more than 24 hours after admission, contact tracing was not done and no prophylaxis was given. The boy was a Year 11 pupil at a local secondary school but he had not attended school since the end of the previous term. However, the boy had met socially with classmates during the holiday. The possibility of meningococcal disease had not been ruled out at this point, and so, in line with national guidance, the head teacher of the school was contacted. A standard letter was circulated to all parents in the school informing them that there had been a case of suspected meningitis.

[‡] This applies to meningitis only; other situations may require the public health doctor to be notified immediately.

**Case study**

**Case B**

Tuesday 5 January

A 13-year-old girl was admitted to hospital with a three-day history of headache, fever, vomiting, photophobia and neck stiffness. She had become unwell on Saturday 2 January, but had attended school on Monday 4 January before being admitted on the Tuesday evening. An initial diagnosis of probable meningococcal meningitis was made, and she was treated with intravenous antibiotics. The public health doctor 'on call'/'appropriate person' was informed, and contacts were traced and given prophylaxis.

**Q When cases are notified 'out of hours', how does 'handover' take place, and to whom? How do you ensure that links between cases are not missed?**

On the morning of Wednesday 6 January, the Consultant in Communicable Disease Control (CCDC)/'appropriate person' was informed of the admission of case B, and identified cases A and B as both attending the same school.

**Q What action would you take at this point?**

The CCDC immediately visited the hospital, interviewed both cases, reviewed the notes and discussed the cases with the respective clinicians. It rapidly became clear that the two cases did not know each other, either at school or socially, did not live in close proximity, and had no known friends in common. Clinically, case A was still considered to be pneumococcal meningitis, whereas case B was now considered to be viral meningitis and the intravenous antibiotics had been discontinued.

**Q What would you do in the light of these findings?**

In view of this, the school head teacher was contacted and informed of the situation. He was advised that, as the second case was now considered to be viral meningitis, there was unlikely to be a link between the two cases, and that no further action needed to be taken. Later that afternoon, the head teacher phoned to inform the CCDC that parents in the school had heard rumours that there were two cases of meningitis in the school, and were starting to panic. He had discussed the situation with the chairman of the school governors, who had requested that the whole school be given antibiotics.

**Q How would you respond to this request?**

The head teacher was advised that, as case A was considered unlikely to be meningococcal meningitis, and case B was considered viral in origin, the administration of antibiotics to the whole school would not be an appropriate course of action. However, a letter was prepared for all parents, informing them of the second case, explaining the difference between bacterial and viral meningitis, and reassuring them that whole school prophylaxis was not necessary.

However, over the New Year weekend, an adjoining local health organisation* had seen several cases of confirmed Group C meningococcal meningitis, of which two school pupils had died. As a result, that health organisation had carried out an extensive school-based prophylaxis and immunisation campaign over the New Year weekend. This had, inevitably, attracted considerable publicity in the local media, and local parents were concerned that their children were not being offered a similar level of protection.

**Q How would this change your management of the situation?**

In view of this, before letters were sent to parents, the regional epidemiologist was consulted and the situation carefully discussed. This was to ensure that the planned course of action was correct in terms of following national guidance, but also defensible, given the public expectations of action. In view of the fact that, by this time, neither child was considered to be suffering from meningococcal disease, and that one child had not attended school for over two weeks, the policy of no further action was supported.

**Q Do you consider this position to be defensible? Would you be satisfied with this response if you were a parent? Who else might have a legitimate interest in ensuring the appropriateness of your 'do nothing' policy?**

In spite of this support, expectations of action were very high. In the ensuing two days, the CCDC was asked to justify the 'do nothing' policy to: the chairman of the school governors, the chairman of the local health organisations, the chief executive of the local health organisations, the Director of Public Health, the local Member of Parliament and a considerable number of parents. All were assured that the situation would be kept under careful review and, should the circumstances change, consideration would be given to further action in the school.

* In this context, the local health organisation was a health authority, but in future may be a PCT or other body responsible for the health of a population greater than a single general practice.

**Case study**

**Case C**

Saturday 9 January

A 15-year-old girl was admitted with a two-day history of fever, headache, vomiting, neck stiffness and a spreading haemorrhagic rash. A diagnosis of probable meningococcal septicaemia was made. The public health doctor 'first on call'/'appropriate person' was notified of the case 12 hours after admission. The CCDC was informed of the case at 8 p.m., when it was realised that this case was a Year 11 pupil at the same secondary school as cases A and B.

**Q Now what would you do? What issues do you have to take into consideration?**

It immediately became clear that the 'do nothing' option was no longer tenable. In public health terms, the two previous cases could have been discounted, as being 'not confirmed meningococcal', and the argument made that there was still only one probable case of meningococcal disease in the school. National guidance would have defended the decision to still do nothing. However, in the eyes of the public, the secondary school had now suffered three cases of meningitis, and we had already refused to act on the first two.

Although the first case was considered by the consultant paediatrician to be pneumococcal disease, the clinical investigations had proved inconclusive. Tests indicated that case A was suffering from a serious bacterial infection but, after five days, blood cultures were negative and the exact causative organism was still not known. This left room for doubt that it might have been due to meningococcal infection. If this had been the case, it would have meant that there had been two cases in the school in a week. This would have been reasonable grounds for offering whole school prophylaxis.

**Q Would you alter your policy now? What action would you consider taking?**

The regional epidemiologist was consulted immediately, and agreed that it would be impossible to defend a 'do nothing' decision in the public arena, and that a whole school antibiotic prophylaxis programme should be offered. It was decided, however, that there was no justification for offering vaccination as no case of Group C disease had been identified.

**Q How and when would you act? What factors would you take into consideration in making this decision?**

Having decided on a whole school programme, it was felt this should be done as soon as possible, and ideally on Monday 11 January. Although it would have been logistically much easier to plan the prophylaxis session on the Monday, and administer it on the Tuesday, it was felt the risk of another case coming to light on the Monday was too great to warrant delaying the programme by an extra day.

**Q Who would you notify? How would you contact them on a Saturday night?**

By this time it was 9 p.m. on a Saturday evening. It was decided the two key players who needed contacting that night were the Director of Public Health (DPH) and the head teacher of the school.

The Director of Public Health was in the process of moving house and was living in temporary accommodation. The hospital switchboard, who kept contact details of all the public health doctors, did not have his new telephone number.

**Q How would you contact a key member of staff if you did not have his/her number? Do you know how to contact all key members of your organisation out of hours? Which members of staff are on a 24-hour call-out rota? Is this sufficient to cope in the event of a major emergency?**

The telephone directory yielded the number of his secretary, but she did not have a note of his telephone number at home. A spark of inspiration led to a call to the local GP in the village, who kindly paid a house call to ask the DPH to phone his CCDC as soon as possible. By 10 p.m., direct contact was made and the situation explained.

**Q How would you contact a head teacher at home on a Saturday evening? How would you contact any other officer of the local authority? Do you know the call-out arrangements for your local authority? Where might you find this information?**

Contacting the head teacher proved equally tortuous. A call to the local authority 24-hour emergency number provided contact numbers for several members of the education department. The Director of Education was able to provide the home telephone number of the head teacher, who was contacted directly, and the situation and proposed action explained.

**Q Once you have made contact, how would you set about planning your prophylaxis session?**

By 11 p.m., the key players were aware of the proposed plan, and an Incident Team Meeting was arranged for 2 p.m. on the following afternoon, at the headquarters of the local health organisation.

**Q Do you know how to gain access to your office at the weekend? Do the telephones work? Are the computers switched on? Is there food and drink available?**

An Incident Team Meeting was convened on Sunday 10 January. Those present at the meeting included:

- the CCDC
- a consultant in public health
- a specialist registrar in public health
- the school head teacher
- the emergency planner from the local education authority
- a school nurse manager
- a microbiologist
- the community pharmacist
- the press officers from the education authority, the local health organisations and the NHS Regional Office.

**Q What additional people would you invite to the Incident Control Team Meeting? How would you contact them out of hours? What arrangements are in place in your organisation for calling out community services staff out of hours? Does the community unit have a 24-hour emergency number?**

For many of the people present there was no official 24-hour call-out system in place, and in many cases successful contact was made only by chance. The community pharmacist was interrupted in the middle of a Sunday League football match! A community paediatrician was unable to attend the meeting but was contacted by telephone and arrangements made for medical support for the school nurses.

**Q What are the main functions of an Incident Control Team in a situation such as this? What decisions have already been made, and what remains to be decided?**

The decision had already been made that antibiotics should be offered to the 1100 pupils at the secondary school, and the purpose of the meeting was chiefly to decide on the logistics of the operation, and to determine the content and mode of publicity.

**Q What would you expect from each member of the Incident Control Team?**

The community pharmacist successfully secured 1100 doses of ciprofloxacin, and the school nurse manager was confident of being able to provide a team of school nurses to administer the antibiotics. The consultant community paediatrician was not able to attend the meeting, but undertook to provide a team of community paediatricians to attend the school as medical support for the nurses and to help with information and counselling to parents.

The head teacher had prepared a roster for each class to ensure the smooth and steady presentation of pupils to the nursing team, so as to disrupt the school day as little as possible. The logistics of the operation were therefore decided upon very rapidly.

**Q What would you consider to be the greatest challenge facing the Incident Control Team? What issues need to be taken into consideration? How would you go about tackling these problems? Who would you turn to for advice?**

The greatest problem lay in the communications. The decision had been taken that the operation should be undertaken without delay. Unfortunately, as the planning was undertaken on a Sunday, with the session planned for the Monday, there was no prospect of sending a letter home to parents to warn them of what was to happen, or to seek consent for their children to be given antibiotics. The community paediatrician suggested that, as the children were 12 years old or older, they should be invited to give their own consent to the administration of the antibiotics, once they had been informed of the situation. This was agreed as the only way forward, given the time constraints. A press release was prepared and agreed, and sent to the local radio station for broadcasting that evening, in the hope that it would reach some parents, and arrangements were made for the CCDC to be interviewed at 7 a.m. on the local radio to publicise the session. It was arranged to post large notices at the school entrance for parents to see at the start of the school day.

**Q How would you deal with queries from the parents? How quickly could your organisation set up a telephone helpline? Who would man it? How many lines would you need? What information would the telephone operators need in order to answer the queries?**

To deal with the anticipated parental enquiries, arrangements were made for a telephone helpline to be set up within the department of public health. Telephones were linked into a 'hunt group' so that additional telephones would not be required, and to allow secretaries within the department to act as helpline operators. The Incident Control Team thus needed to prepare press releases, letters for students to inform them of what prophylaxis they had been given, letters to pass onto their GPs, letters informing parents if prophylaxis had not been given, and a question and answer sheet for the helpline operators.

**Q What else could go wrong? Are your major incident plans robust enough to deal with an escalating incident?**

During the course of all the preparations, the public health doctor on call/'appropriate person' was notified that two ten-year-old children had been admitted to hospital with suspected meningococcal septicaemia. Both children attended the primary school sharing the same campus as the 'outbreak' secondary school. The secondary school site occupied two buildings, on either side of the primary and nursery school. The secondary school children walked through the primary school campus six or seven times each day, and interacted with the younger children.

**Q Now what would you do? Is there any further action that you need to take? If so, what, when and by whom?**

In view of this development, the regional epidemiologist advised that all children on the campus should be offered prophylaxis. This would involve offering measured doses of rifampicin syrup to 600 primary school children and 100 children at the attached nursery school. As parental consent would be required for these younger children, and as it would take some time to acquire, measure and bottle 700 doses of rifampicin syrup, it was decided that the primary/nursery school prophylaxis session should be held on the Tuesday, to allow time for the arrangements to be made and for letters to be sent out. The primary and nursery school head teachers were contacted that evening, the situation explained, and arrangements were made for a planning meeting to take place on the following day.

At 9 p.m., while the letters for the secondary school were being typed, the local health organisation's computer file server automatically shut down.

**Q Are you confident that your communications systems are sufficiently robust to cope with a major incident? Does your computer system have an automatic closedown at night? Do your mobile phones work within the building? Do you know where the mobile phone 'blackspots' are in the local vicinity? How would you cope in the event of a power cut?**

On Monday 11 January, 1100 secondary school children were offered antibiotic prophylaxis during the course of the school day. As a result of the meticulous planning by the school, the programme was completed before the end of the school day, and each class suffered a maximum of 20 minutes disruption to their daily routine. There was intense media interest, and as a result of the lack of advance warning to parents, the department of public health received in excess of 150 telephone calls during the day from parents seeking information about the day's events.

On Tuesday 12 January, 700 primary and nursery children received rifampicin syrup at school. As parents had received advance notice, there were no phone calls received by the department, and very few personal queries on the day.

The week after the prophylaxis session, a structured debriefing session was held, to which all participants were invited. This allowed all those who had been involved to discuss the management of the incident, their role in it, and to identify both good and bad points that could be addressed in the Major Incident Plan.

# Key issues

## Notification

The Public Health (Control of Disease) Act 1984, sections 10, 11 and 12, describe the process of notifying a notifiable disease.[1] Section 11 states: 'If a registered medical practitioner becomes aware, or suspects, that a patient whom he is attending within the district of a local authority is suffering from a notifiable disease or from food poisoning, he shall ... send to the proper officer of the local authority ... a certificate ...'

Section 10 of the 1984 Act, and Regulation 3 of the Public Health (Infectious Diseases) Regulations 1988, give a list of the diseases which are required to be notified.[2] A 'notifiable disease' is simply a disease which appears in that list. In order to notify such a disease, a certificate has to be completed in writing, and sent to the 'Proper Officer' of the local authority.

The 'Proper Officer' is the person who has been appointed by the local authority as being the correct or proper person to receive that information. The local authority may appoint the Chief Environmental Health Officer to be the 'Proper Officer', but most local authorities nominate the Consultant in Communicable Disease Control (CCDC) of the local health organisations to receive the notifications.

There are four main reasons for notifying a disease.

- To trigger action. This may be urgent, such as closing down a restaurant to contain an outbreak of food poisoning, or identifying close contacts of a case of meningitis.
- To maintain a watching brief on rare illnesses to identify outbreaks. Hepatitis A and leptospirosis are examples.
- To monitor and evaluate the effectiveness of immunisation programmes – for example, for measles, mumps, diphtheria and pertussis.
- To monitor the international spread of disease such as cholera, typhoid and viral haemorrhagic fever.

For monitoring disease incidence, sending a certificate to the Proper Officer will suffice. However, to trigger immediate action, this process is not fast enough. It needs to be supplemented by, but not replaced by, a direct telephone call to the local 'appropriate person'. Not all notifiable diseases need to be notified urgently, but meningitis and food poisoning are two of the most common diseases that need a rapid response.

---

**Exercise 2.1**

- Read Part II of the Public Health (Control of Disease) Act 1984. Apart from the definitions of notifiable diseases, there is a great deal of fascinating material about what you can, and cannot, do if you have a notifiable disease.

- Ensure that you know where to find or obtain notification forms, and where to send them.

- Consider which of the notifiable diseases you should report by telephone. If you were the CCDC, which ones would you like to hear about 'out of hours'?

- Ensure that you know how to contact your local department of public health and the CCDC at all times and the 'appropriate person'. There is a public health doctor on call, 24 hours a day.

---

## Investigations

One of the key problems with meningitis is that it is difficult to diagnose. In the early stages of meningococcal septicaemia, the symptoms may appear like a non-specific flu-like illness. Not all patients with meningococcal septicaemia get the characteristic 'tell-tale' rash. Not all patients with clear meningitic symptoms have meningococcal disease. Many have viral meningitis: a few may have pneumococcal meningitis.

Unfortunately, there is, as yet, no foolproof, near-patient test which will give a reliable and rapid answer. In the face of considerable uncertainty, the public health doctor has to decide on a course of action which may have a profound effect on the community, and will rely to some extent on laboratory results to help in making the decision. Laboratory tests may be very non-specific, such as the C-reactive protein (CRP) test, which may suggest severe infection, but gives no clue as to the causative organism. Levels of this protein rise to 10–40 mg/L when there is mild inflammation or a severe viral infection. Levels of 40–200 mg/L suggest acute inflammation or bacterial infection, while levels may rise to over 300 mg/L in severe bacterial infections. Perhaps the biggest problem with the CRP test is that it is time sensitive. The levels begin to rise six to nine hours after the onset of infection, and peak at 48 hours. Levels then drop rapidly over the next 48 hours and are likely to have returned to normal after a week of illness. Normal levels in a person with a slowly evolving infection may therefore be misleading.

Some tests are very specific, such as blood culture. Culturing *N. meningitidis* from a sterile site such as blood or CSF is usually considered the 'gold standard' for diagnosis, but these sites are often sterile if pre-admission antibiotics have been given and, even if the culture is positive, the result may not be available for several days. Modern molecular techniques, such as the polymerase chain reaction (PCR) test, may be very sensitive, but may be negative even in severe disease. This test detects and amplifies meningococcal DNA, but as it uses a very small sample of blood, it is possible for that small sample not to contain any DNA to amplify. This could result in a PCR which is reported as negative, even when the blood culture is eventually found to be positive.

Serology is very accurate, but is of no practical use in the incident as it requires acute and convalescent paired serology to allow interpretation, and the result may not be available until several months after the event.

Throat swabs may be positive in up to 50% of cases and the swab is likely to remain positive even if pre-admission antibiotics have been given. The meningococcal strain identified may be assumed to be the same as the invading strain, and meningococcal strains isolated from throat swabs of household contacts are also likely to be the same as the case strain, especially if the index case is a child. Taking throat swabs from family members before giving prophylaxis may help to identify the causative organism. However, this does require great sensitivity and such a request should always be accompanied by counselling, as a positive result may engender feelings of guilt. Transmission between family members is a two-way process, and it is not possible to distinguish who first picked up the organism.

Public health doctors rely heavily on the clinical impression of the admitting doctor. If the clinical impression is that the patient is likely to have meningococcal infection, then a diagnosis of a 'probable' case is made, and public health action may be triggered. This may involve the giving of prophylaxis to contacts of cases, or the distribution of a letter to school. If, however, the diagnosis is equally likely *not* to be meningitis, then the diagnosis of a 'possible' case is made. Public health action is likely to be postponed in this instance, until the diagnosis becomes more clear cut.

---

**Exercise 2.2**

- Discuss with your local clinicians and the laboratory which tests they use to establish the diagnosis of meningitis. How long do the tests take to give a result?

- Discuss with your local clinicians what factors they take into consideration when making the decision to inform the CCDC of a 'possible' or 'probable' case of meningococcal infection.

- Find out from your local CCDC what proportion of reported 'meningitis' cases are finally confirmed. Are the proportions the same for both children and adults?

# Dealing with uncertainty

When meningococcal infection occurs in a school-age child, the head teacher must be informed as soon as possible, with the parent's consent, and kept fully 'in the picture'. This will include sharing with the head teacher any uncertainties about the diagnosis. When dealing with anxious parents, and even press enquiries, the CCDC and head teacher must work closely together, and can be powerful allies, providing mutual support. However, this demands mutual trust and understanding about the difficulties and uncertainties of the illness, and its effect on the school community. Although the head will rely on the professional judgement of the CCDC in deciding the appropriate course of action, s/he will welcome being involved in the decision-making process. In the case of a single school child being affected, national guidelines are clear, and are usually accepted as 'best practice'. However, in more complex cases, where national guidelines cannot be prescriptive, the head teacher will appreciate a reasoned discussion of possible courses of action.

In this case, the head teacher and the school governors were, understandably, alarmed by the tragic events in the neighbouring district, and were anxious to ensure their pupils were as well protected as possible. In refusing their demands for whole-school prophylaxis at this point it was vital to ensure that they fully understood the principles behind meningococcal prophylaxis to reduce the risk of linked cases, and the risks inherent in giving widespread medication. Parents also need access to this sort of information, and it can readily be provided in the awareness-raising letters to parents to advise them of a case in a school.

From the point of view of professional 'security', making difficult, and often unpopular, decisions should not be undertaken alone. Senior colleagues and local, regional and national experts are always available to assist in deciding upon the most appropriate course of action. Far from being seen as a sign of weakness, the head teacher will be reassured to know that you have asked for expert advice, and will be able to pass this confidence on to parents and governors.

---

**Exercise 2.3**

- Read the national guidance: 'Control of meningococcal disease: guidance for consultants in communicable disease control'.[3]
- Draft a letter which a CCDC might send to a school informing it of a case of meningococcal disease. Does it contain all the information you would like to receive as a parent?
- Ask your local CCDC for a copy of the letter sent to schools, and compare it with yours.
- Read the national guidance: 'Management of clusters of meningococcal disease'.[4]

# Communication

Most public health emergencies require a multi-agency response.[5] The precise agencies and individuals involved will vary according to the incident, and the key to a successful outcome is communication. Breakdown in communication both within and between agencies has been repeatedly cited as the major cause of escalation of small incidents into larger ones, and of public criticism of an otherwise well-handled incident. Communications with the public and the media are equally important, and the successful handling of the public relations aspect of an incident is as important as its professional management.

The successful management of an incident very often stands or falls by the standard of the communication that takes place. Similarly there may be a wide gulf between the professional evaluation of how well an incident was managed, and the public perception of what actually happened, if the public relations aspects of the incident were poor. For the local health organisations, in most instances, communication *is* the incident.

To be successful, communication needs to be accurate, relevant, directed at the appropriate audience and, above all, timely. No matter how well presented the information, it will be of little value if half the people who needed to know do not receive it, or receive it two days late. It can sometimes be difficult to judge who exactly needs to know. In the case of a school meningitis case, the issue of patient confidentiality is of central importance, and this is particularly so when the media become involved. The pupil should never be named, and the parents should be notified that, even though the school is to be informed, confidentiality will be absolutely maintained. It is almost inevitable that family, friends and neighbours will become aware of the diagnosis, and that the name of the index case may appear to become public knowledge. However, this should never be taken at face value, and great care must be taken not to confirm what may only be a suspicion or a lucky guess on the part of the media or other parents.

Perhaps the biggest problem with communication is ensuring that it is disseminated rapidly enough. There will always be criticism that information was delayed. It is as well to request the help of as many people as possible in preparing press statements, briefings for public health colleagues, question and answer sheets for helpline operators, letters for parents and any other information that is required. The single biggest advantage of holding an Incident Control Team Meeting is that information can be given to as wide a range of people as possible, in the shortest possible time. It is the most efficient information-sharing mechanism available. An added advantage is that not all members of the team will be public health professionals, and they can act as 'lay readers' of any public information material that you produce.

The most serious communication problem faced during this incident was the inability to contact the parents of the school children on a Sunday evening.

Contacting the health professionals, and representatives from the education authority, proved surprisingly straightforward overall. Only the public health doctors were part of a 24-hour call-out rota, and so other professionals were co-opted onto the team according to their availability. However, it was probably easier to find people at home on a cold Sunday in January than it would have been on a warm Sunday afternoon in June. The availability of staff on this occasion probably owed more to luck than to the robustness of the major incident plan, and this issue was addressed as one of the 'lessons learned' at the debriefing session.

To let the parents know our intentions, a number of methods were used. Initially, on Sunday evening, a press release was sent to the local radio station, with the request to broadcast details of the prophylaxis session during the course of the evening. Unfortunately, Sunday evening was recognised by the radio station as having low listener figures, and it was felt that few parents would hear about the session by that route. Arrangements were also made for an interview on the morning news programme at 7 a.m., and it was felt this was more likely to reach a large audience. Large notices were posted at the school entrance to inform parents and children, but it was anticipated that many children would make their own way to school, and parents would not see the notices. At the time of this incident, very few school children carried mobile phones, and therefore using these to contact parents was not an option. This might be a useful route to parents now. A considerable number of phone calls were received during the day, indicating that many parents did hear about the session 'on the grapevine', although the 'grapevine' can be a considerable problem when rumours begin to spread. In difficult circumstances it can prove an invaluable mechanism for spreading information. It can be used proactively by asking parents to tell as many other parents as possible, so that the news is spread like a 'cascade' or 'snowball'.

---

**Exercise 2.4**

- Apart from parents, it is vitally important to keep the local GPs informed of events. Find out from your local CCDC how GPs are contacted out of hours. How does the Chief Medical Officer communicate urgently with all GPs using the 'Public Health Link'?

- Find out how to contact key members of other organisations on a 24-hour basis. How would you contact your local authority, regional epidemiologist or national experts on a Saturday night?

- What other organisations know how to contact you out of hours?

- Who would you contact at the local radio station or newspaper if you needed to make an urgent announcement?

# Consent

In view of the very short timescale, and the difficulty in contacting parents, it was decided that children should be invited to give their own consent for the antibiotics, once they had been informed of the situation. Although this method had been used before, mainly for screening programmes, it was considered as a method of 'last resort' for the administration of medicines. As the school in question was a secondary school, it was clear that most of the older children would be 'competent' to give their own consent. School staff identified all those children who they felt could not be expected to self-consent, and their parents were contacted by telephone to obtain consent. Any child who declined antibiotics was given a letter advising his/her parents of the fact, and suggesting that they could see their GP if the child should later change his/her mind. If any child suffered from a pre-existing medical condition, or was on any medication, his/her GP or hospital consultant was contacted for advice before antibiotics were given.

Those parents who did phone the school or the telephone helpline were unanimous in their support of the action that had been taken. Given that they had been kept informed of the unfolding situation in the previous week, they appreciated the changing circumstances. In view of the events in the neighbouring local health organisations they were grateful that action was under way, whereas in other, less anxious circumstances, they may have been more critical of the decision. This was not an easy decision to make. It is not always the correct decision, and it is advisable to discuss the circumstances with the defence societies before making the final decision.

---

**Exercise 2.5**

- Find out what is meant by 'Gillick competence'.[6] Explore with your local paediatricians, both hospital and community based, what factors they take into account in deciding a child's competence to consent to treatment.

---

# Debriefing

During the course of a major incident, it is easy to be disheartened by the apparent chaos. In the relief that follows the 'stand down' after any major incident, it is easy to believe that it all went well. It is extremely valuable to view the management of the incident objectively, shortly after the event, to identify what can be learned from the successes and failures. A structured debriefing session to which all participants are invited is a useful tool. There will be many aspects of the management of the incident that went well, and the team should be congratulated on those elements. There will be certain elements that did not go so smoothly, and these should be honestly identified so that the major incident plan can be improved. In any major incident, systems, rather than people, fail at critical points, and these must be identified to prevent a repetition. In this incident, the major strength was identified overwhelmingly as the teamwork and the mutual support that all team members enjoyed. A number of weaknesses were identified, the most obvious being communications: with the public, with other members of staff on a Saturday night, and electronically.

Where possible, these problems have been addressed. The computers in the public health department no longer switch off automatically at 9 p.m.

# Key definitions

## Consultant in Communicable Disease Control (CCDC)

The CCDC is a doctor, trained in public health, microbiology or infectious diseases, who is responsible for the prevention and control of communicable disease within a defined population. This defined population was previously that of the district health authority, but following changes within the health service, the CCDC is usually now responsible for the population of a number of primary care trusts through what will become the Health Protection Agency (HPA) (*see* Further reading, DoH 2002). The role of the CCDC is wide ranging and has been evolving rapidly to encompass a number of health protection issues. The chief functions of the CCDC are:

- to undertake the surveillance of communicable disease
- to act as an information broker within the community on issues relating to communicable disease
- to develop policies and guidelines to ensure the effective management of communicable diseases
- to investigate outbreaks and incidents of communicable disease, and to ensure control measures are put in place to prevent further cases
- to maintain a community perspective on cases of communicable disease
- to act as the 'Proper Officer' of the local authority for the purpose of notifications of infectious diseases
- to co-ordinate the health service response to non-infectious environmental hazards, including acute chemical incidents
- to participate in the emergency planning function of the health service, especially in relation to protecting the health of the public, and to providing public information in the event of an emergency.

Other roles which may be undertaken by CCDCs include:

- acting as the District Immunisation Co-ordinator for childhood and adult immunisation programmes, e.g. the annual flu immunisation programme.
- participating or leading on the provision of health services for homeless people and asylum seekers.

## Regional epidemiologist

The regional epidemiologist is a doctor, usually with a background in communicable disease control, who works at the level of the government regional office. The role is chiefly to co-ordinate the surveillance of disease across a number of smaller districts, and to act as a source of expert advice and additional support to CCDCs who are dealing with a complex incident, or one which crosses a number of district boundaries. The regional epidemiologist will ensure that incidents which have major implications for use of resources or for media interest are brought to the attention of the Regional Director of Public Health and/or the Department of Health.

## References

1  The Public Health (Control of Disease) Act 1984. Command 22. DHSS, London.

2  The Public Health (Infectious Diseases) Regulations 1988. SI 1456. DHSS, London.

3  PHLS Meningococcal Infections Working Group and Public Health Medicine Environmental Group (1995) Control of meningococcal disease: guidance for consultants in communicable disease control. *Communicable Disease Review Report.* **5**(13): R189–R195.

4  Stuart JM, Monk PN, Lewis DA, Constantine C, Kaczmarski EB, Cartwright KAV *et al.* (1997) Management of clusters of meningococcal disease. *Commun Dis Rep Rev.* **7**(1): R3–R5.

5  Department of Health (1998) *Planning for Major Incidents. The NHS Guidance.* DoH, London.

6  *Gillick* v *West Norfolk and Wisbech Area Health Authority* [1986] AC112, [1985] 3 All ER 402, [1985] 2 BMLR 11 (HL).

## Further reading

- Hawker J, Begg N, Blair I, Reintjes R and Weinberg J (2001) *Communicable Disease Control Handbook.* Blackwell, Oxford.
- Chin J (2000) *Control of Communicable Disease Manual* (17e). American Public Health Association, Washington, DC.
- Department of Health (2002) *Getting Ahead of the Curve (a strategy for combating infectious diseases – including other aspects of health protection).* DoH, London.

## Useful websites

- Public Health Laboratory Service: http://www.phls.co.uk.
- UK Department of Health: http://www.open.gov.uk/doh.
- National Meningitis Trust: http://www.meningitis-trust.org.uk.
- Meningitis Research Foundation: http://www.meningitis.org.

# CHAPTER 3

# Towards evidence-based healthcare: practical issues in getting research into practice

## James Munro

## Introduction

There is widespread agreement that evidence-based healthcare is a 'good thing', and should be encouraged at every opportunity. There is also a great variety of research evidence available about effective and ineffective treatments, diagnostic techniques, preventive measures and so on. However, despite all this evidence, there is also much healthcare activity which remains ineffective, and much uncertainty about how best to use the research evidence which we do have in order to influence everyday practice.

This chapter is about the practical business of how to go about 'getting research into practice', so that more of what is done is at least influenced by good quality evidence. In this chapter we take the evidence as given – in other words, there is no discussion here of how evidence is created, sought, summarised and appraised. Some of these issues are covered in Chapter 9.

## Learning objectives

- To identify the range of issues involved in implementing practical programmes of evidence-based change.
- To appreciate some of the obstacles to achieving such change, and ways in which they might be tackled.
- To be aware of the range of implementation tools and techniques which are available.

## What is the problem?

It is now widely understood that simply publishing the results of research will, in most cases, have no effect on practice at all. In part, this is because there is simply far too much research for anyone to keep abreast of new findings – even if they didn't have anything else to do, like seeing patients or running the NHS. However, there are many other reasons why research findings may be difficult or impossible to implement, which will be explored through the case studies in this chapter.

The problem of getting research into practice is certainly not a new one. When James Lind, a naval surgeon, conducted what is thought to be the world's first randomised controlled trial in 1747,* the results showed fairly convincingly that 'the most sudden and visible good effects were perceived from the use of the oranges and lemons', rather than any of the other treatments dispensed (though the sample size of 12 sailors was rather small by modern standards). However, it was not until 1795 – almost 50 years later – that the Admiralty was moved to action, issuing an order to keep generous supplies of lemon juice on board naval vessels. Scientific confusion, Lind's low status in the medical profession and the costliness of fresh fruit all contributed to the delay. Of course, we come across very similar issues in implementing research findings today.

In many ways, the task of getting research evidence into practice is really just one particular case of the general problem of achieving change in any complex organisation such as a health service. As other chapters in this book indicate, the NHS, like healthcare systems in other developed countries, is characterised by complex structures and rules, ambiguous and contested goals, multiple competing interests, diverse financial arrangements, high fixed costs, scarce resources, and different cultures and even languages among its different tribes. In such an environment, it is not surprising to find that research evidence is only one – and far from the most important – of many influences on action.

## Case studies in promoting evidence-based care

### The FACTS project

We established the FACTS (Framework for Appropriate Care Throughout Sheffield) project in Sheffield specifically to address the practical question of how to achieve evidence-based changes in clinical behaviour across a whole community of doctors – in this case, all general practices in the city. The key objective of the project was to help general practices deliver more effective care.

We felt that this could best be achieved by running a series of specific 'change programmes' which were both evidence-based and in line with health service priorities.[1] Each change programme would draw together coalitions of key people committed to achieving a particular change, determine in detail how the change might be achieved and what obstacles might be encountered, and use a

---

* James Lind (1753) *A Treatise of the Scurvy in Three Parts, Containing an Inquiry into the Nature, Causes and Cure of that Disease, Together with a Critical and Chronological View of what has been published on the subject*. Published by A Millar, London.

wide range of interventions with practices to initiate and support the change.[2] An important part of the FACTS philosophy was that appealing to professional pride and a sense of good medical practice would be more likely to generate sustainable change than simply bullying or coercing doctors to move in a particular direction.

We selected potential change programmes for further development following consultation with clinicians, managers and others, and after considering the range of criteria listed in Box 3.1. Our first two change programmes focused on interventions for cardiovascular disease: aspirin for the secondary prevention of heart attack, and anticoagulation in patients with atrial fibrillation for the primary prevention of stroke. In practice, as we shall see, these two programmes turned out very differently.

---

**Box 3.1:  Criteria for judging potential programmes in general practice**

- Is the issue common enough to warrant the effort and locally relevant?
- Are significant health service resources involved?
- Is the proposed change clearly defined?
- Is there good evidence to support the change?
- Can the likely barriers be overcome – at least in theory?
- Can the effects of a change programme be determined?
- Will the programme enhance collaboration between practices – or at least not hinder it?

---

**Case study 1: aspirin**

*The evidence for change*

There is much good-quality evidence to show that aspirin is effective in reducing the risk of heart attack or stroke in those who are at high risk – that is, those who have previously suffered from one of these conditions, or have a history of transient ischaemic attack, angina or angioplasty.[3] Given that the cost of aspirin is so low (about £1 per patient per year), it is clear that daily treatment for those at risk is likely to be both cost-effective, compared to many other interventions, and easily affordable for the NHS.

However, only about two-thirds of those who could benefit from this treatment receive it, suggesting that there is plenty of scope for improving matters.[4]

*The planned change*

The aim of the aspirin programme was to ensure that all patients at high risk of heart attack or stroke were taking aspirin daily, apart from those with a contraindication. The programme was supported by good-quality evidence, and might potentially lead to worthwhile health and resource gains. In addition, the costs of change were likely to be low, both in terms of the costs of aspirin itself, and the time and effort involved on the part of practices. The planned change was clearly defined, and did not need the involvement of other agencies in order to succeed.

---

### Exercise 3.1

- How would you go about promoting this change, in practical terms?
- Think of the steps that are needed: what difficulties do you anticipate?
- How would you evaluate the success of the programme?

---

### Case study 1

*How we went about it*

The process of developing the programme began with exploring the views of key players – GPs, health authority commissioners, consultants, local academics – on the desirability of the change, and what the obstacles and opportunities might be. The point of such discussions was both to inform the design of the programme and also to raise the issue of aspirin prescription and awareness of the forthcoming programme, in order to create some sense of anticipation.

Commonly, such exploratory discussions are held in groups or committees brought together for the purpose. However, against received wisdom, we felt it would be better to speak to people individually in order to allow them to express their views and reservations openly and without having to take up a position in relation to other key players. This proved to be very successful and was appreciated by our interviewees.

These discussions identified a number of potential obstacles to the change we were trying to achieve. The most important was the concern by practices that they would find it difficult and time-consuming to identify their high-risk patients not already on aspirin. Some practices believed that they had already 'done' aspirin and felt that all those who might benefit were already on treatment.

Given these concerns, and in the light of our wider reading on approaches to changing practice,[5] we designed an 'aspirin pack' for use by practices who signed up to the programme. The pack had a strongly practical focus and was modelled on the sorts of materials drug companies use to promote their products. It included a manual on how to carry out the programme, a summary of the research evidence supporting it, a leaflet for patients, stickers and bookmarks for patient notes, administrative materials, and coasters, pens and mugs with an 'I ♥ aspirin' slogan, to stimulate interest and discussion.

The pack was carefully designed in order to minimise the effort involved on the part of practices that wished to implement the programme, and to allow practices to be flexible in how they carried it out. Rather than dictate 'this is how you should implement the evidence', the philosophy of the pack, and the wider programme, was to say 'here's a range of ways in which you can move closer to using the evidence'.

At the consultation stage, practices had been worried about how to identify the patients who should be on aspirin. Although many practices ran computer systems which they used for patient registration, repeat prescribing, routine letters and so on, they did not know how to use their systems to find particular kinds of patient – for example, those with a diagnostic code of coronary heart disease, or those who were being prescribed a nitrate or digoxin. To address this barrier, we developed simple search strategies that could be used with each of the main GP computer systems, and offered participating practices informal IT training for their staff, ranging from simple advice to group or individual tuition. Providing this support and encouragement to practices became a major part of the job of the FACTS practice worker.

This practical support enabled practices to identify the patients who might benefit from aspirin, while at the same time developing their skills and confidence in using the computer to support evidence-based care. Of course, it also provided practices with an incentive to take part in the programme, and allowed us to monitor how they were progressing.

*What happened*

The aspirin programme was launched by means of a short announcement at a local continuing medical education event, at which a respected local clinician was speaking. Again imitating the tactics of drug companies, further information on the programme, and a display of the materials used, were set out in a stand. Twenty-seven practices registered their immediate interest in the programme, and these contacts were followed up by the practice worker.

Over the following months similar displays were set up at other events being run for primary care teams. Eventually, over two-thirds of the 102 practices in the city had joined the programme. As each practice registered its interest, it was contacted by the practice worker and an initial meeting arranged to discuss the programme and address any concerns. After this, each practice was supported to undertake the programme in the way that suited it best. The emphasis here was on adapting to the practice's own style and way of working, and offering only as much help as the practice wanted.

*Programme outcomes*

Did the programme succeed? In total, 68 practices signed up to the programme, of whom seven later dropped out. At least 44 practices completed the programme, with the remainder getting some way through it. Most practices needed between one and three visits from the practice worker in order to complete it.

In terms of prescribing, ongoing audit showed that over 2500 high-risk patients were started on aspirin as a result of the programme, more than 80% of whom continued to take it in the long term. Quantitative analysis of PACT (*see* Chapter 1, p. 46) data showed that aspirin prescribing by programme participants tended to increase at a greater rate than by non-participants (or by practices in neighbouring districts) over the period of the programme. This difference was sustained for at least nine months after the programme ended. Using the published research data on risk reduction,[3] we estimated that the programme might have prevented about 50 cardiovascular events per year.[6]

The programme also appeared to be a success in the eyes of participants. Qualitative evaluation of the programme showed that participants had been motivated to join because they saw it as 'good clinical medicine', and 'it looked as if it would be very easy to implement'.[7] Interviews with participants also made it clear that they valued the independence of FACTS from both the formal management structures of the NHS and from drug companies, both of which were regarded with some suspicion. Practices appreciated the practical support along with the sense that they were joining a wider community of practices trying to improve their care. Crucially, GPs tended to see the FACTS team as 'on our side', and 'not being out to get us'.

## Case study 2: anticoagulation

By contrast, the second of the planned change programmes did not go so well.

*The evidence for change*

At least six randomised controlled trials have assessed the effects of anticoagulation with warfarin on stroke risk in patients with non-valvular atrial fibrillation.[8] The evidence so far suggests that warfarin may reduce ischaemic stroke risk substantially (by around 60%), while introducing a small increase of haemorrhagic stroke risk. Aspirin also reduces stroke risk, but by a smaller amount (about one-fifth).

Despite the convincing evidence that exists, and the emerging consensus that anticoagulation should be considered in all patients with atrial fibrillation, only about one in seven of those with this indication and no contraindications receive therapy.[9] Thus, just as with aspirin, this is an area ripe for a change programme.

*The planned change*

The main purpose of this programme was to increase the prescribing of warfarin to patients with atrial fibrillation who were at high risk of stroke. At the time of the programme, much anticoagulation was managed in specialist clinics provided by the local hospitals, which were already struggling to meet demand. Adding to their workload did not seem like a good idea, especially since there was emerging experience, and some evidence, suggesting that anticoagulation could be safely managed in primary care settings, which would be more convenient for patients. We therefore aimed to encourage general practitioners to initiate and monitor the anticoagulation of patients in their own surgeries.

**Exercise 3.2**

- How would you go about promoting this change, in practical terms?
- Think of the steps that are needed: what difficulties do you anticipate?
- How would you evaluate the success of the programme?

**Case study 2**

*How we went about it*

As before, we began by exploring the views of key stakeholders – general practitioners, hospital physicians and health authority staff – on the desirability and feasibility of the proposed change. In contrast to the aspirin programme, this involved not simply a discussion about the evidence and how to implement it routinely, but also a series of very involved discussions about the different ways in which anticoagulation services could be provided and paid for.

*What happened*

The suggestion that anticoagulation services might be better provided in primary than in secondary care settings met with objections from many quarters. In a qualitative evaluation of the programme, we identified the range of barriers perceived by those involved:[10]

- disinvesting from existing providers
- lack of information on activity and costs
- uncertainty over the quality and safety of proposed new services

- concern about increasing workload in general practice
- diversity of views within general practice
- difficulties in communication
- lack of leadership.

From the viewpoint of many general practitioners, the idea of initiating and monitoring anticoagulation in primary care seemed like being asked to take on somebody else's work without payment. One GP commented: 'Maybe the nurses could do it, but they are already working to full capacity.'

Directing resources into a new primary care service inevitably raised questions about whether funding could be withdrawn from the existing secondary care service – a solution popular with GPs but, understandably, not with the hospitals. The health authority found itself taking the flak. 'The GPs see us as incompetent but actually they need educating about financial issues,' one health authority manager argued. 'They have no idea about the difficulties of withdrawing and fixed costs. The reality is that we could easily end up paying twice.'

There were also questions about whether the service would be safe – mainly from the hospitals, though they also acknowledged that the quality of the existing service was unknown: 'Within the hospital it's so fragmented that we have no quality control.'

Very quickly, the whole programme became bogged down in argument about where anticoagulation services should be provided, who was doing the work now, how it should be funded, and so on. The longer discussions continued, the further we seemed to get from a clear and unambiguous evidence base.

Eventually, we decided to go ahead with a programme focused simply on supporting general practitioners in identifying patients for whom anti-coagulation might be indicated, and helping them initiate the therapy – regardless of the debate about whether this constituted a new service or should attract additional funding. Our approach was very similar to that of the successful aspirin programme: clear comprehensive materials, practical help and plenty of moral support.

*Programme outcomes*

In the event, only a small number of practices joined the anticoagulation programme, of which only six returned monitoring figures allowing the impact of the programme to be assessed. The figures showed that 88 patients on digoxin and with a high risk of stroke had been identified who were not anticoagulated. However, when reviewed, 35 patients were not in atrial fibrillation when examined, and a further 30 had a contraindi-cation to warfarin or declined to take it. In the event, only four patients were newly started on warfarin – a very disappointing outcome after months of planning, discussion and practice support.

Exercise 3.3

- Why did the anticoagulation programme fail where the aspirin programme had succeeded?
- What range of factors should be considered?
- Which, if any, of these could have been tackled in practical ways?
- How might this change programme have been tackled differently?

# Some reflections on getting research into practice

Implementing research evidence seems often to be seen as a technical task (use the right tool) or as a managerial one (tell people what they should do). By contrast, our experience in the FACTS project over a number of years has strengthened our belief that evidence-based change must begin from a position of clear understanding and respect for practitioners.

The *understanding* that is required includes an understanding of the situation of practitioners, the constraints and incentives they face, and the cultures – both the 'macro' professional and the 'micro' practice cultures – which shape the nature of workable solutions.

The *respect* involves a recognition that almost all in the healthcare system are already 'trying to do their best', are busy and tired, and have seen a lot of change before. Though, like anyone, healthcare professionals have a range of motivations for what they do, effective change strategies should recognise that a powerful one is the desire to practise well: to do good work.

## The nature of the change

The nature of the specific change practitioners are being asked to make is clearly central to how likely it is to occur. In the case studies above, there are sharp contrasts between the two programmes in terms of the clarity and complexity of the changes proposed. In the case of aspirin, the research evidence was unambiguous, the clinical decision making involved for any given patient was relatively simple, there was no significant resource implication (whether financial, staffing or workload) and no need to involve other agencies in the change. Prescribing aspirin to patients at risk just made 'clinical sense'.

However, in the case of anticoagulation none of these conditions applied. The evidence was still, to a degree, contested and even if accepted did not lead to straightforward clinical decisions either for doctors or patients.[11] In addition, increasing the number of patients requiring anticoagulation would have effects – on other services and the flow of funds – which went far wider than a single practice.

Of course, as soon as proposals for change threaten the interests of one or more groups, whether through loss of status, role or resources, resistance is bound to result, and may often prove decisive, irrespective of the merits of the evidence.[10]

---

**Exercise 3.4**

- Think of an evidence-based change to practice you would like to promote locally.
- Where does it fall on the spectrum of clear–ambiguous? Simple–complex?
- Could it be made clearer? Simpler?
- Whose interests are threatened by your change?

---

## The approach to change

Those trained in the arts of 'evidence-based medicine' and 'critical appraisal' soon come to feel the evidence speaks for itself. They forget that, to the rest of the world, it does not – and that in fact the source, the shape, the support and the stories about proposals for change are very often far more important than 'what the evidence says'.

The source of the message should be a trusted one, and this may require the source to be independent of the financial and managerial structures and interests of the formal healthcare system. In FACTS, we were fortunate to be supported by, yet outside, the local structures of the NHS and to have a respected working general practitioner in a central role. There was a clear sense among local practices that FACTS understood the everyday problems of primary care, was 'on their side' and had no other conflicting interests.

Building support for proposals in advance of making them public is clearly helpful, especially if the support comes from those who themselves inspire trust. There is much literature on the importance of 'opinion leaders', though we found that the support of an opinion leader seemed less important to practices than knowing who else – which colleagues – had already signed up to a programme. Clinicians, like everyone else, may give greater weight to what their peers are doing than to what 'a paper, somewhere' says.

Some thought should be given to the 'shape' of messages about evidence-based change, so that they are suited to their audience. In dealing with general practices, which are used to a series of short, intensive encounters with patients, we found that brief, clear, practical communications worked well.[2]

In addition, in most cases there is no reason why promoting the use of evidence has to result in fixed solutions, so we focused on flexible programmes which would allow practices to opt in to as much or as little as they felt able to manage. Although the evidence may dictate the 'what', it ought to be possible to leave the 'how' to clinicians. Allowing flexibility in implementing the evidence isn't some kind of compromise; it simply accepts the reality that, whatever rules you may think you have set down, people themselves must decide when and how they apply. This is inevitable, and the advantage of accepting it is that you create more opportunities to bring practice closer to an evidence base.[12]

It is well recognised that the stories people hold in their heads, and share with others, are also powerful in determining how they react to evidence on particular interventions. For example, in the case of anticoagulation, personal or even second-hand experience of an adverse effect may be enough to induce strong resistance. In a recent study, one GP said: 'I lost a patient as an SHO, so that puts me off warfarin.'[13]

Conversely, experience of not having treated a patient who might have benefited is also a powerful motivator. In the same study another GP noted: 'I actually had two 50-year-olds who had strokes from atrial fibrillation because they didn't get warfarin ... that really hit me.'

Of course, as an evidence promoter you can't 'get rid of' the stories people have, because they are intrinsic to being human. However, you can try to discover what the stories are – so you can understand the barriers to your proposals. You can also pass on new stories (truthful ones!) which might support the changes you are trying to make: for example, 'Practice X started this programme last week and they are really pleased with the results already.'

## Tools and techniques for getting research into practice

There is a wide range of techniques and tools which you may find helpful in thinking practically about getting research into routine practice (*see* Box 3.2). All of these techniques have been subject to evaluations, and each has its own strengths and weaknesses, so the choice of which technique or tool, if any, to deploy is a matter of understanding the situation clearly.[5]

In general, the research evidence available on the effectiveness of these approaches in changing clinical practice leads to a number of conclusions. First, although financial incentives are powerful in changing behaviour, they may produce unpredictable and possibly unwanted results.[14] Second, relatively simple and discrete behaviours, such as the ordering of tests or prescribing

---

**Box 3.2: Some tools and techniques used in promoting evidence-based practice**

- Clinical audit.
- Guidelines and protocols.
- Computer-assisted prompts, reminders and decision aids.
- Continuing professional education/development.
- Administrative/environmental changes.
- Feedback systems.
- Resources, support or financial incentives.
- Peer assessment or review.
- Opinion leaders.
- Educational outreach ('academic detailing').
- Decision aids for patients.
- Coalitions of interest.

---

medicines generically rather than by the pharmaceutical company brand name, are the easiest to change. Third, by implication, more complex areas of clinical practice such as consultation skills, clinical management of chronic conditions or referral to other agencies are much more difficult for any single intervention to alter; and, of course, the ability to define what constitutes evidence-based practice in such areas may be much more difficult too. Fourth, and perhaps predictably, those clinicians most likely to respond to programmes of evidence-based change tend to be those who are already closest to the agreed standard of good practice.

---

**Exercise 3.5**

- Think of an evidence-based change to practice you would like to promote locally.
- Which – if any – of the tools and techniques set out above might be helpful in this situation? Why?

---

# Conclusions

While there is much talk of research and development in healthcare and public health settings, thought and action has been so strongly weighted towards research, and so little towards 'development', that we have few clear ideas about what development even means. The recently increasing interest in 'implementation' of research findings often tends to give the impression that this is a technical task, so that if we could simply deploy 'effective interventions' – like guidelines or financial incentives – then we could cure the 'sick' (non-evidence-based) clinicians.

The reality, as I have tried to show, is different and inevitably messy. Getting research into practice is highly context-specific and a solution that works in one place may fail in another – just as, in healthcare, not all patients respond to the same standard treatment. In both situations there is a range of effective interventions available, and success lies in first understanding the problem, and then tailoring a solution to fit as well as possible.

# References

1 Hodgkin P, Eve R, Golton I, Munro J and Musson G (1996) Changing clinical behaviour on a city-wide scale: lessons from the FACTS project. *Journal of Clinical Effectiveness.* **1**(1): 8–10.

2 Eve R, Golton I, Hodgkin P, Munro J and Musson G (1997) *Learning from FACTS.* ScHARR Occasional Paper 97/3. School of Health and Related Research, University of Sheffield, Sheffield.

3 Antiplatelet Trialists Collaboration (1994) Collaborative overview of randomised trials of Antiplatelet therapy I: prevention of death, myocardial infarction and stroke by prolonged Antiplatelet therapy in various categories of patients. *BMJ.* **308**: 81–106.

4 Campbell NC, Thain J, Deans HG, Ritchie LD and Rawles JM (1998) Secondary prevention in coronary heart disease: baseline survey of provision in general practice. *BMJ.* **316**: 1430–4.

5 Eve R, Golton I, Hodgkin P, Munro J and Musson G (1996) Beyond guidelines: promoting clinical change in the real world. *Journal of Management in Medicine.* **10**: 16–25.

6 Hodgkin P, Eve R, Golton I, Munro J and Musson G (1999) *An Aspirin a Day ... Final Report of the FACTS Aspirin Programme.* Centre for Innovation in Primary Care, Sheffield.

7 Musson G (1996) *Qualitative Evaluation of the FACTS Aspirin Programme.* Sheffield Business School, Sheffield.

8 Hart RG, Benavente O, McBride R and Pearce LA (1999) Antithrombotic therapy to prevent stroke in patients with atrial fibrillation: a meta-analysis. *Annals of Internal Medicine.* **131**: 492–501.

9 Bungard TJ, Ghali WA, Teo KK, McAlister FA and Tsuyuke RT (2000) Why do patients with atrial fibrillation not receive warfarin? *Archives of Internal Medicine.* **160**: 41–6.

10 O'Cathain A, Musson G and Munro J (1999) Shifting services from secondary to primary care: stakeholders' views of the barriers. *Journal of Health Services Research and Policy.* **4**:154–60.

11 Devereaux PJ, Anderson DR, Gardner M, Putnam W, Flowerdew GJ, Brownell BF *et al.* (2001) Differences between perspectives of physicians and patients on anticoagulation in patients with atrial fibrillation: observational study. *BMJ.* **323**: 1218–22.

12 Tanenbaum S (1993) What physicians know. *New England Journal of Medicine.* **329**(17): 1268–413.

13 Freeman AC and Sweeney K (2001) Why general practitioners do not implement evidence: qualitative study. *BMJ.* **323**: 1100–2.

14 Iliffe S and Munro J (1993) General practitioners and incentives. *BMJ.* **307**: 1156–7.

# Further reading

## Books

- Dunning M, Abi-Aad G, Gilbert D, Hutton H and Brown C (1999) *Experience, Evidence and Everyday Practice: creating systems for delivering effective health care.* King's Fund, London.
- Greenhalgh T (2001) *How to Read a Paper* (2e). BMJ Books, London.
- Trinder E and Reynolds S (2000) *Evidence-based Practice: a critical appraisal.* Blackwell Science, Oxford.

## Papers

- Grol R, Dalhuijsen J, Thomas S, in 't Veld C, Rutten G and Mokkink H (1998) Attributes of clinical guidelines that influence use of guidelines in general practice: observational study. *BMJ.* **317**: 858–61.
- Isaacs D and Fitzgerald D (1999) Seven alternatives to evidence-based medicine. *BMJ.* **319**: 1618.

## Websites

- Netting the Evidence: http://www.nettingtheevidence.org.uk. An extensive and well-organised resource of UK and international websites on various aspects of evidence-based healthcare.
- National Electronic Library for Health: http://www.nelh.nhs.uk/. A new and growing resource which brings together many high-quality sources of evidence-based guidance.

# Acknowledgements

Ros Eve, Paul Hodgkin, Gill Musson and Ian Golton were the driving forces of the FACTS project and the work described here is theirs. I'd like to thank them for their valuable advice on writing this chapter.

# CHAPTER 4

# Working across agencies that impact on health and healthcare

*Frances Cunning*

## Introduction

This chapter focuses on the issues involved when health organisations work in partnership with other organisations and agencies whose actions have a direct and/or indirect effect on the population's health. It provides pointers to achieving a successful outcome of partnership activity.

Working in partnership towards integrated planning as a means of improving health and reducing inequalities in health is a key component of current government policy in the United Kingdom. Professionals in public health have long been involved in developing partnerships. Internationally, a key example is the World Health Organization's Healthy Cities initiative.[1] Nationally, a prime example is the development of the Health Action Zone (HAZ) work.[2] Both of these activities have assisted in building infrastructures for many areas of partnership working.

The health status of a population and the individuals it comprises depends on a wide variety of factors (*see* Chapters 5, 6 and 8). Health organisations cannot achieve health improvement without working closely with a wide variety of voluntary and statutory agencies. Developing collaborative relationships through partnership working is the modern approach to creating interventions designed to improve the population's health.

## Learning objectives

By working through this chapter the reader should be able to:

- identify the key stakeholders and partners to provide effective public health action

- appreciate the relevance of different organisational cultures in influencing public health practice
- understand the different levels involved in partnership working with other organisations and agencies
- understand the importance of working with colleagues from different professional and organisational backgrounds in order to improve health
- identify the skills and mechanisms required for effective working with other organisations and agencies.

# Definitions

The World Health Organization definition of *Health for All 2000* encapsulates the importance of cross-agency working.[3]

> '*Health for All* requires the co-ordinated action of all sectors concerned. The health authorities (and now primary care organisations) can deal only with part of the problems to be solved and multi-sectoral co-operation is the only way of effectively ensuring the prerequisites for health, promoting health policies and reducing risks in the physical, economic and social environment.'

The publication of *Health of the Nation*, the first attempt at developing a health strategy for England, provided a major boost for collaborative working.[4] It acknowledges that delivery of the strategy requires close working relationships between a wide range of departments and agencies at national and local level. These 'healthy alliances' were defined as 'a partnership of individuals and organisations formed to enable people to increase their influence over the factors that affect health and well-being – physically, mentally, socially and environmentally.'

In the United Kingdom, since the 1970s, monies have been made available in each health community for jointly funding the commissioning of projects and services by the health services and the local authority, for client groups whose needs make demands common to health and local authorities, e.g. older people and people with mental health problems. Expenditure has been agreed between all partners, including the voluntary sector. Since the 1998 Health Act there has been greater flexibility for pooling resources between local authorities and the NHS.[5] Previously, the different financial systems of these two organisations and the associated legal issues have made agreement and implementation of joint funding extremely difficult.

Working across organisations and agencies to improve health outcomes has been variously called collaborative working, joint working, multi-agency working or a partnership. Partnership is generally used to mean agreed working arrangements between organisations, formally recognised by the organisations concerned. Some partnerships are governed by legally binding contracts. These may include agreements and timescales relating to decision making, membership, numbers required for a quorum and the amount of delegated and spending power. Such agreements are detailed in the partnership's terms of reference. Joint working and multi-agency working refer to a less formal approach. Collaborative working is defined as working in combination.

Common to all these approaches are shared values, common goals and resources.

Because working in partnership is often a difficult task and generally expensive in terms of people and time, we need to be sure that there is added value from adopting this approach.

As a rule, public health professionals and agencies are expected to respond appropriately to political pressure and government imperatives. These may not necessarily equate to local health priorities as determined through health needs assessment. This is illustrated by the case study used in this chapter. However, the response to political imperative in relation to health must integrate the demands of the government with the needs of the local population. This is the delicate balancing act, which, if successfully executed, epitomises effective public health practice, and a positive outcome for everyone involved.

# The key components of successful collaborative work

There are eight key components to take into account in ensuring successful collaborative work for health improvement. These are as follows.

## 1 The purpose of collaborative working

The purpose of collaborative working is to solve problems. Some health problems are complex and difficult and require a multidisciplinary, multi-agency approach. Others do not.

The first question to ask is: 'Do we need to work jointly to solve this problem and to achieve a positive change?'

If it is accepted that joint working is required, it is essential that, at the earliest stage, there is an explicit and common understanding of what partnership means and agreement to working in this way.

In developing partnership working the following issues need to be taken into account.

- How to demonstrate the added value of working together.
- The agreement of a common purpose to guide the partnership is required. This is generally achieved by jointly identifying and agreeing the aims and objectives which will inform the strategic development. To do this, work needs to be done in creating a common vision. This can be supported by consulting

widely with all the relevant stakeholders, organisations, users of services, carers and support groups.

---

**Exercise 4.1**

- What criteria should be considered in determining whether there is added value in partnership working on a particular project?
- Identify a group with which you have been involved. Comment on its cohesiveness and commitment to achieving a common task. How do you know when a group is or is not cohesive?
- Describe the added value of partnership working. Illustrate your answer with an example from your own experience.

---

## 2 Setting up the partnership

It is essential to create and implement the appropriate processes in order to ensure a successful outcome to partnership work. Effective processes ensure successful outcomes.

There is a series of stages to consider in setting up a partnership, as follows.

- Developing a cohesive group, fully committed to the task.
- Mechanisms for communicating the issues involved so that the relevant individuals and organisations have a clear and unequivocal understanding of what is required.
- Achieving the right balance of people involved to include the relevant competence and level of seniority necessary for joint decision making.
- Obtaining formal agreement to establish a particular partnership, including joint resources, work plans and delivery mechanisms.
- Obtaining support for the work. Identify the key influencers who will shape the proposals appropriately and who will act as champions for the outcomes.
- Developing governance arrangements for the partnership needs to be outlined. This will include the terms of reference for the main partnership and any substructures. Lines of accountability also need to be determined and agreed.
- Agreeing mechanisms for conflict resolution.
- Identifying the cultural, structural and resource requirements and developing plans to resolve these.
- Identifying the required outcomes needed as a focus for the partnership.
- Identifying and agreeing mechanisms for decision making.
- Processes and governance arrangements need to be put in place and time spent on building trusting relationships.

Exercise 4.2

- You have been asked to create a new partnership group. Describe the steps which you would take to ensure a successful enterprise.

## 3 Identifying leadership for the partnership

Partnerships require the appropriate leadership. The leader should be skilled and experienced in partnership work, be able to motivate and influence people, and get the best out of what will always be a diverse group. S/he must achieve a positive outcome through using the people comprising the partnership. They will only do this if they trust and respect their leader (*see* Chapters 8 and 10).

The leader will need to:

- develop an action plan based on the shared vision, aims and objectives and measure review and evaluate progress
- develop the group, build trust and positive relationships
- work at the pace of the group and pay constant attention to where the group is in respect of both task and process maturity
- encourage decision making, especially where the decisions are difficult.

Exercise 4.3

- There are a variety of leadership theories which have been developed to explain different leadership styles and approaches. Describe the main leadership theories currently in vogue. Choose one leadership theory and describe how this can be effective within a partnership-working framework.
- Identify two leaders you have encountered in your work who have different leadership styles. Describe their leadership styles and how this affects work achievement.

## 4 Driving the work

It is important to identify the key drivers underpinning any piece of work or project. These will include the following.

- Political imperative.

- Source of problem identification, i.e. by the community, through health needs assessment, by a lobbying pressure group.
- Personal/organisation ambition. There may be someone in a particular organisation who has a passion to change some aspect of health or an organisation's vision may be focused on a particular issue. In either case, the ambition may be far removed from community perceptions and needs.

---

**Exercise 4.4**

- There are a variety of factors which drive people to accomplish given tasks. Identify these factors and discuss how they may be harnessed to achieve a desired outcome. Use examples from your own experience to illustrate your discussion.

---

## 5 Communication

It is essential to remember that people working together in partnership mode come from different backgrounds and use different language to express themselves. Additionally, professions and disciplines have their own languages allowing them to communicate more efficiently. However, the language of one profession will be meaningless to others. In order to communicate well, the following points need to be taken into consideration.

- Avoidance of 'jargon' or language which is profession/discipline specific, e.g. medical or social work terminology.
- Creation of a group norm which allows people to feel comfortable enough to ask for an explanation when they do not understand.
- Development of communication mechanisms within and across the partnership, e.g. are there formal minutes? Will there be a newsletter? How will the group communicate its decisions? Will it be appropriate to use email?
- Consider the use of glossaries for explanations of common terminology.

---

**Exercise 4.5**

- Describe a group which you have worked with. Discuss its communication processes. How would you improve communication in the group and between the group and other groups?
- Effective communication requires trust, openness, honesty and clarity of thought. Discuss this in relation to your own experiences.

---

## 6 Resources

The partnership will need to manage its resources and to acquire additional resources when needed. A system needs to be created for resource management.

> **Exercise 4.6**
>
> - Finance is only one resource required to achieve a successful outcome in partnership work. Describe what other types of resource are essential to support partnerships and their specific contribution to outcome.

## 7 Involving communities

Involvement of the voluntary and community sector, patients, carers and the public is a key expectation placed on public organisations.

Mechanisms need to be identified to ensure full involvement of the relevant communities and how the work of the partnership is communicated to engage the local population.

> **Exercise 4.7**
>
> - Involvement of local communities is a vital component of partnership working. How would you work towards effective community consultation and participation in solving a health issue?

## 8 Evaluation and review

Appropriate monitoring and evaluation processes need to be established to ensure the partnership is achieving its objectives.

Members of the partnership need to agree a mechanism for this process.

> **Exercise 4.8**
>
> - A partnership group has asked you to present a paper to them outlining an evaluation and review system for their use. Describe how you would accomplish this task. What key areas would you pay attention to before presenting the report to the group?

# Summary

Partnership working is a delicate flower. Like a flower, it needs constant nurturing, watering and feeding, pruning and training. If, in the end, despite all efforts, the partnership is incapable of achieving success, then it should, as with a dying plant, be consigned to the compost heap and a fresh start made.

The following case study illustrates how the eight key components are applied in a real life situation.

---

### Case study

**Developing an integrated approach to addressing the health of asylum seekers in the Canalside area**

### Background

The Immigration and Asylum Act 1999 (UK) led to the dispersal of asylum seekers throughout the country to relieve pressure on London and the South East of England.

This legislation prevents asylum seekers from joining their natural communities in areas of the United Kingdom. Therefore, instead of areas volunteering to take asylum seekers on an *ad hoc* basis, all areas have been informed they will receive a regular intake dependent on the numbers of asylum seekers entering the country and the dispersal rates.

The Home Office expected a consortium to be established in each health region of the country comprising representatives from local authorities, the police and the health sector (in Canalside's region, two representatives from the health sector drawn from sub-regional areas). The remit of this group is to negotiate and liaise with the Home Office on issues concerning asylum seekers being sent to the region and ensure the numbers identified for each area are communicated to local authority staff.

There is also a sub-regional group with membership drawn from the local authorities in the area, the police, accommodation providers, large voluntary agencies such as the Red Cross and one public health specialist (PHS) representing all the local health authorities. The remit of this group is similar to that of the regional group and includes the co-ordination of issues affecting the placement of asylum seekers at a sub-regional level.

### Canalside

Canalside is a city of roughly 500 000 inhabitants, of which approximately 6% are from black and ethnic minority communities. Unusually for a city, the black and ethnic minority communities are not confined to any particular area or ward, nor do they congregate in the inner city. They are spread around the periphery of the inner-city area. The city has above average levels of deprivation and unemployment, with all the associated mortality and morbidity rates. The sub-region in which Canalside is situated comprises four urban areas. Canalside is twice as large as the next largest urban area.

Over the years there have been a number of asylum seeker and refugee communities arriving in the city with some good examples of partnership working to help meet their needs and ease the demand on services. In addition Canalside has a good track record of working in partnership at a number of levels, with particularly strong working links between the primary care organisations and the local authority. This has been significantly refined and strengthened by the current administrative approach to developing high-level partnerships in each local authority area.

The same public health specialist has led on all of this work from the health perspective. This continuity helps to build good practice, develop thinking and ideas over time and invariably cut down the time required to begin delivering outcomes. However, the negative aspect of this includes the history and quality of relationships and processes an individual brings to a piece of work. These may affect how that individual is perceived – either as a capable practitioner who delivers or someone who does not.

### Issues affecting the health of asylum seekers

Services are likely to have varying levels of experience in dealing with new arrivals and they are often woefully ill-prepared to meet need. In addition, some specialised services may be concentrated in or around London and not available locally, e.g. legal professionals specialising in immigration.

Traditionally, health communities have responded to immigrant demands based on work done in the 1950s and 1960s and it is the Consultants in Communicable Disease Control who have taken prime responsibility for this area of health service provision. There has been a focus on screening for infectious disease such as tuberculosis, hepatitis and, latterly, HIV and AIDS. This approach, which reflected the dominant philosophy of the day, was understandably concerned with protecting the health of the resident population.

There are a number of issues that impact on the health of asylum seekers which are not a threat to the resident population. These include:

- the original reason for seeking asylum
- the whole experience of seeking asylum
- isolation both of cultural dislocation and language
- housing
- material needs and the voucher scheme
- racism and discrimination
- prospects for employment.

These factors may lead to social and economic exclusion that is detrimental to health. There is a need to take a more holistic approach to deal with the problems being experienced by this diverse group.

The challenges to the health service include:

- a lack of outreach services except for some aspects of communicable disease control, e.g. tuberculosis and health visitor management
- conflicts between differing health belief systems
- a lack of appropriate community infrastructures, which may affect development of community approaches
- the underdevelopment of interpreting services
- the issue of local health services being the only agency responsible for all asylum seekers but not being in control of the arrivals in the area.

The immediate issues with which the health services are concerned include:

- explaining the NHS system
- providing access to primary care
  - registering with a GP
  - emergency treatment
  - getting a prescription
  - registering with a dentist
- access to screening services
  - TB and other infectious diseases
  - health-visiting links
- access to mental health services
  - counselling
  - specialised trauma counselling
- access to secondary care services
  - predicting pressure points
- building capacity of the voluntary and community sector to provide support
- interpreting services.

### The problem

As the issues affecting Canalside, the largest urban area, were dominating the meetings of the sub-regional partnership, the public health specialist employed by the local primary care organisations felt that more specific joint working across all the relevant agencies was required. In order to achieve this, the public health specialist had to link all the individual organisations dealing with the issues, work with others to find pragmatic solutions and work towards common ownership of the issues and contributions to the solutions.

One of the immediate tasks undertaken by the public health specialist was to make links with other key agencies in Canalside (particularly the local authority and private accommodation providers). The rationale for this was to acquire information about the location of asylum seekers and to register them with local general practitioners. The public health specialist's experience of working with previous groups of asylum seekers had illustrated the importance of access to primary care. Part of this problem was persuading the accommodation providers to actively support asylum seekers to register with local general practitioners.

A group comprising representatives from a number of health organisations was established to resolve local problems in the health service and to deal with issues of service configuration. One of the functions of the group was to enable information sharing and to reassure health workers that they were not alone in dealing with this diverse group of people. A significant amount of time was spent in proactively working with groups of practice managers to ensure that general practitioners' lists were not closed to the asylum seeker, i.e. asylum seekers were able to register with local GPs. In some areas of Canalside, all new arrivals were registering with one particular practice as a result of information received from fellow asylum seekers. Working with practice managers ensured that the workload was shared and that everyone had the same information about which accommodation providers were using the areas and the numbers of asylum seekers expected. Key information included access to interpretation services. Building up access to these services included working with primary care organisations to enable them to understand the needs of asylum seekers and to ensure they had access to healthcare. Primary care organisations were encouraged to increase funding for interpretation and enable these services to be extended to dentists and opticians.

An opportunity arose to pursue funding for a nurse consultant post. Although the group was not fully established with an agreed work plan, everyone knew the most important health issue was to sort out access to primary care and it was considered appropriate to apply for this funding. The bid was successful and a nurse consultant for asylum seekers is now in post.

The group does not exist in isolation. The local authority had a group to enable internal co-ordination. In addition, there was a local community forum in Canalside that involved the voluntary groups who worked with refugee and asylum-seeker communities coming into the area. The forum had particular difficulty in influencing statutory agencies as it was not well organised.

This forum provided an opportunity to create a Canalside-wide group. This facilitated the development of an informal partnership for involving local consumers in decisions about the way services should be provided. It also enabled statutory services to respond to the voluntary agencies and the individual communities about local service provision. The public health specialist now chairs the forum that comprises representatives from health, the local authority, the police, voluntary sector agencies and from the different communities. However, this is not a strategic group and it has acted mainly to provide a place for information exchange, with representatives alternating at each meeting. It has not set direction and more thought needs to be given to its future evolution.

Despite this, by the end of 2001 there had been significant strategic discussion on the following issues which enabled a work programme to be established:

- whether there should be a centralised location for the initial assessment or prompt linkages to local primary care services
- how to deal with communication of information about individual health issues and whether the records should be hand-held
- what diseases were common in the countries of origin
- finding solutions to such practical problems as the provision of interpreters for GPs who have no appointment system
- development of mental health services, especially cross-cultural counselling services for men
- provision of services which involve a number of agencies, e.g. play workers.

**Success**

The successes are listed as follows:

- development of a local partnership
- effective communication with accommodation providers and other agencies
- effective communication with regional and sub-regional agencies
- securing interpreting services
- working with primary care to support those practices most under pressure
- building links with dentists
- securing funding for a nurse consultant
- securing additional funding for TB screening
- training conferences and seminars for professionals and the voluntary sector
- working on a sub-regional basis to develop mental health services capacity
- using asylum seekers as a resource
- supporting the development of community groups, community development and establishing an accredited course for volunteers working with asylum seekers
- supporting health impact assessment on policy and initiating action.

Exercise 4.9

- You have been asked to set up a partnership group to support asylum seekers from an African country. What factors would you need to take into account before creating the group? What are the key steps you would take in setting up the group? How would you know if your partnership group was working well? How would you tell if things were not going well? How would you rescue a failing group?

- Apart from physical and mental health issues, what factors must be taken into account in providing for asylum seekers? Why would a partnership approach help you to provide an effective service for asylum seekers?

# References

1 World Health Organization (2002) *Healthy Cities Make a Difference*. www.who.dk/eprise/main/who/home.

2 Department of Health (1997) *Health Action Zones Invitation to Bid*. Circular EL(97)65. DoH, London.

3 World Health Organization (1985) *The WHO Declaration of Health for All 2000*. WHO, Copenhagen.

4 Department of Health (1992) *The Health of the Nation*. DoH, London.

5 Department of Health (1998) *Health Act*. DoH, London.

# Further reading

## Partnership working

- Audit Commission (1998) *A Fruitful Partnership: effective partnership working*. A management paper. Audit Commission, London.
- Department of Health (1998) *Partnership in Action: new opportunities for joint working between health and social services*. A discussion document. DoH, London.
- Department of Health (1999) *Health Action Zones: learning to make a difference*. DoH, London.
- Ewles L and Simnett I (1999) *Promoting Health: a practical guide* (4e). Baillière Tindall, London.
- Fieldgrass J (1992) *Partnerships in Health: promotion collaboration between the statutory and voluntary sectors*. Health Education Authority, London.
- Home Office (2002) *The Partnership Standard for DATs. Quality Standards for Managing Programmes to deliver the National Drugs Strategy*. Home Office, London.

- Naidoo J and Wills J (1998) *Health Promotion Foundations for Practice*. Baillière Tindall, London.
- NHS Executive (1998) *Unlocking the Potential: effective partnerships for improving health*. NHS Executive, Leeds.
- NHS Executive (1998) *Working in Partnership with Voluntary Organisations and Communities*. NHS Executive, Leeds.
- Pratt J, Plamping D and Gordon P (1998) *Partnership Fit for Purpose*. King's Fund, London.
- Pratt J, Gordon P and Plampling D (1999) *Working Whole Systems*. King's Fund, London.
- Wakefield HAZ (2001) *Health Action Zones in Yorkshire and Humber: advancing together for health*. Wakefield Health Authority, Wakefield.
- Wilson A and Charlton K (1997) *Making Partnerships Work*. Joseph Rowntree Foundation, York.

## Leadership

- Birkenshaw J and Crainer S (2002) *Leadership: the Sven Göran Eriksson way*. Capstone Publishing Limited, Oxford.
- Capper SA, Swayne LE and Ginter PM (2001) *Public Health Leadership and Management*. Sage Publications Ltd, Thousand Oaks, CA.
- Dilts RB (1996) *Visionary Leadership Skills*. Meta Publications, CA.
- Koller J, Zaleznik A, Badaracco J and Farkas C (1998) Leadership. *Harvard Business Review*.

## Asylum seekers and their issues

- Aldous J, Bardsley M, Daniell R *et al.* (1999) *Refugee Health in London*. East London and the City Health Authority, London.
- Audit Commission (2000) *Another Country Implementing Dispersal Under the Immigration and Asylum Act 1999. Audit Commission Briefing*. Audit Commission, London.
- Elders in Exile, a Report from the Northern Refugee Centre (1995).
- Levenson R and Coker N (1999) *The Health of Refugees*. King's Fund, London.
- Mahmoud A, Gray P and Wakeling D (2000) *Mental Health Care for Refugees and Asylum Seekers*. The Mental Health Foundation, London.
- World Health Organization (1996) *Mental Health of Refugees*. WHO, Geneva.

# CHAPTER 5

# Developing health programmes and services, and reducing inequalities

## *John Cornell*

## Introduction

This chapter is in three sections. Section 1 looks at differences in health between individuals and between communities. It goes on to consider what determines whether a particular difference is regarded as an acceptable variation or an inequality. Section 2 looks at the concept of health needs assessment (HNA) in a community as a prerequisite for identifying inequalities and the development of programmes to address them. Having reached this point, Section 3 discusses how choices have to be made concerning which programmes to implement. This involves identifying available resources and making decisions concerning their allocation, accepting the fact that the total needs are likely to outstrip the available resources. Therefore, decisions will have to be made that are likely to limit the provision of services. Some form of framework is required that allows such rationing decisions to be made as fairly, transparently and consistently as possible.

Exercises can be found at the end of each section and points to consider in tackling them can be found at the end of the chapter.

## Learning objectives

- Understand the concept and dimensions of inequalities.
- Understand the factors contributing to the emergence of inequalities.
- Understand methodologies for assessing health needs and identifying inequalities.
- Understand the methodologies for strategy development/action planning.
- Understand the factors influencing the need for rationing.
- Understand the elements involved in making decisions about resource allocation.

# Section 1: Identifying variations and inequalities

Why does life expectancy or mortality from specific conditions such as heart disease vary for people in different parts of the world?[1-8] Why does life expectancy or mortality from specific conditions such as heart disease vary for people in different parts of the same country or different parts of the same county, town or ward?[9-14] To quote from the Acheson Report – the Independent Inquiry into Inequalities in Health: 'Although in general disadvantage is associated with worse health, the patterns of inequalities vary by place, gender, age, year of birth and other factors, and differ according to which measure of health is used.'[15] The purpose of this chapter is to look at a number of issues integral not only to understanding this situation but also doing something about it, from within the NHS.

Variations in death rates within the population are graphically demonstrated in Tables 5.1 and 5.2. Despite a gradual decline in death rates across the whole population in people under the age of 64 years, both tables show differences between the social classes, between men and women and the widening gap over time.

The health of an individual is determined by the interaction between his/her personal characteristics and the environment. The health of the population is the sum of the health of the individuals within that population and is usually described by statistics of mortality and morbidity for that population (*see* Chapter 1). The public health function is aimed at maximising the health of the whole population. Therefore questions of variation in health are fundamental concerns of public health.

**Table 5.1:** European standardised mortality rates per 100 000 population by social class, men aged 20–64, England and Wales, selected years

| | Year | | |
| --- | --- | --- | --- |
| *Social class* | *1970–72* | *1979–83* | *1991–93* |
| I – Professional | 500 | 373 | 280 |
| II – Managerial and technical | 526 | 425 | 300 |
| III(N) – Skilled (non-manual) | 637 | 522 | 426 |
| III(M) – Skilled (manual) | 683 | 580 | 493 |
| IV – Partly skilled | 721 | 639 | 492 |
| V – Unskilled | 897 | 910 | 806 |
| England and Wales | 624 | 549 | 419 |

*Source*: Independent Inquiry into Inequalities in Health Report (the Acheson Report).[15]

**Table 5.2:** Age-standardised mortality rates per 100 000 people by social class, men and women aged 35–64, England and Wales, 1976–92

| All causes | Women (35–64) | | | Men (35–64) | | |
|---|---|---|---|---|---|---|
| | 1976–81 | 1981–85 | 1986–92 | 1976–81 | 1981–85 | 1986–92 |
| I/II | 338 | 344 | 270 | 621 | 539 | 455 |
| III(N) | 371 | 387 | 305 | 860 | 658 | 484 |
| III(M) | 467 | 396 | 356 | 802 | 691 | 624 |
| IV/V | 508 | 445 | 418 | 951 | 824 | 764 |
| Ratio IV/V : I/II | 1.50 | 1.29 | 1.55 | 1.53 | 1.53 | 1.68 |

Source: Harding S, Bethune A, Maxwell R, Brown J (1997).[10]

*Personal characteristics*, such as age and sex, clearly cannot be changed. Genetic factors are currently not amenable to change, though this is likely to happen in the future. Personal behaviours are open to influence, both at the stage where new patterns of behaviour are developing and once behaviours are established. Perception of self and self-confidence also affect our health status.

*Environmental characteristics*: many different aspects of the environment affect our health. These include:

- *Upbringing* – the way in which we are nurtured both pre-and post-natally and how we are subsequently brought up is known to affect health in later life.[16]
- *Education* – the quality, length of schooling and academic achievement have an independent role in determining health in adulthood as well as being related to future employment prospects and levels of income.[3,17,18]
- *Housing* – cold, damp and unfit housing is associated with poor respiratory health as well as it being demoralising to live in poor housing conditions.[19–23]
- *Nutrition* – access to affordable healthy food, cooking skills and knowledge of healthy diets are all known to be important for health.[24–29]
- *Exercise* – regular exercise has a number of health benefits including reductions in blood pressure, weight loss and increased mobility.[30–32]
- *Poverty* – both absolute income levels and low incomes relative to higher incomes within the community/country have an adverse effect on health.[2,33–39]
- *Unemployment* – unemployment is an independent risk factor for poor health as well as its association with other indices of deprivation.[40–47]
- *Social capital* – a number of different dimensions of life have been shown to be associated with poor health, including lack of trust, fear of danger, lack of social networks and lack of involvement with neighbours or community.[48–49]
- *'Physical environment'* – safety, air pollution and environmental noise all have adverse effects on health.[50]

In a sense, all of us are vulnerable to the prospects of poor health. Illness is not a respecter of persons. It is understood and accepted that some people become ill and that others escape. However, there is also a recognition that not all differences or variations in health experience are caused by genetics or quirks of fate and a number of theories have been proposed in explanation.[1,51–53] Many of the factors that influence a person's health are known to be remedial. Thus, differences caused by such factors may be said to be inequitable and unfair.[54]

# Inequality, variation and equity

*Variations* or differences in health are inevitable. Each of us is unique. We have different genetic make-ups, different personalities, different constitutions, characters and experiences. However, where differential overexposure to factors that adversely affect health or, conversely, underexposure to factors that benefit health have given rise to these differences in health, then they can be said to be inequitable. Variations in health are evidenced by differences in morbidity and mortality between people and populations. Such variations raise questions about fairness and justice and require investigation to determine the cause of the variance.

*Equity* concerns the individual being treated fairly and justly and being given the opportunity to attain his/her full potential for health. It is also about ensuring people are helped to take full advantage of the opportunities they have.

*Equality* is concerned with applying equity to everyone.

*Inequalities* are avoidable variations, and therefore unacceptable. To quote from the Government's document *Tackling Health Inequalities – consultation on a plan for delivery*:

> 'Some differences in health status are unavoidable, the consequences of genetic and biological differences in individuals. Many are avoidable, and often unjust. Such inequalities in health are a consequence of significant differences in opportunity, in access and in material resources, as well as differences in personal lifestyle choices.'[55]

## Reducing inequalities

At first sight it seems self-evident that there is a case for intervening to reduce inequalities. However, separating inequality from variation, identifying and agreeing an appropriate intervention and turning this into practical policy and action raise a number of dilemmas. Does a fair distribution of resources mean that everybody should be given an equal amount of money to spend on their health or should resources be allocated according to need? In which case, who defines need? From what and whose perspective should need be considered? Will intervening in one dimension create more inequity in another?

These difficult questions do not let us off the hook. We are required to answer the *key* questions:

- To what extent is a particular variation avoidable and thereby unfair and inequitable?
- Are there known interventions that, if implemented, could change the situation and cause the differences to disappear or diminish?

These questions apply equally to decision making in the clinical management of patients and also to commissioning decisions determining the local provision of healthcare services.

Methodologies for further enquiry into these questions are considered in Section 2. Action planning to address inequalities is touched on in Section 2 but is dealt with in more detail in Chapter 6.

---

**Exercise 5.1**

- List the factors that may be involved in the development of variation in people's experience of health and health services.
- Which of these could be classed as inequitable?
- What theories have been proposed to explain variations in health?

---

**Exercise 5.2**

- Using your own knowledge and local health statistics and information, identify specific examples of variations in health and in service provision in your area.
- Apply the two *key* questions to your chosen example *or* to an example of differences in:
  - mortality or morbidity
  - clinical decision making
  - access to healthcare/'postcode' services (*see* Section 3).
- Choose one of the identified inequalities and devise an action plan or strategy to tackle the issue. What factors should be taken into account? (*See* Chapter 6.)

# Section 2: Health needs assessment

Health needs assessment (HNA) is regarded as the basis for rationally planning healthcare services.[56,57] This emphasis stems from the assumption that by using routine data, applying statistics from research studies or by conducting local research through surveys and questionnaires the local health problems and the number of people suffering from them can be ascertained. Local service provision can then be planned rationally based on an analysis of this pooled information. However, defining and assessing need is much more complex than the logic of the process just described might indicate. This will become apparent as we look at the different facets contributing to an understanding of HNA.

## Defining need, want or demand

Understanding what constitutes need is problematic because it depends from whose perspective it is defined. Patients, health professionals, politicians and the 'well' public have different understandings according to their own particular circumstances. Is it the patient, pressure groups, health professionals, government or society who determine the definitions and whether services will be provided to satisfy them? For example, surveys conducted among doctors, NHS managers and the public, in which they have been asked to rank certain treatments in terms of priority, demonstrate wide disagreements in the order these groups place certain interventions.[58-60] Such surveys uncover the underlying tensions in disentangling the concepts of need, want or demand and translating them into service provision. A flavour of these tensions is reflected in Bradshaw's taxonomy of health need.[61]

Need has also been defined as the 'capacity to benefit'.[62] In the introduction to the text, Stevens and Raftery draw a distinction between the need for health and the need for healthcare. This latter term indicates the use of preventive or treatment services to remedy health problems. The need for health, on the other hand, may go beyond the boundaries of what healthcare services usually provide. For example, improved health may result from the provision of better housing or a job, and so on.

Unfortunately, defining need as 'capacity to benefit' does not help quantify need or clarify its relationship with service provision. From whose perspective is capacity to benefit defined and what sort and how much 'benefit' constitutes benefit? The concept of the QALY (Quality Adjusted Life Years)[63-66] and other measures[67,68] have been devised to try to quantify benefit. Costing health gain allows comparison with other interventions for other conditions. Although superficially attractive, these approaches have a number of drawbacks.[69] Other paradigms of need include Bradshaw,[70] Maslow's 'hierarchy of need'[71] and the 'iceberg' of disease described by Hannay.[72]

Need can also be considered from a number of other perspectives. These include:

- geography – defining a population to investigate
- gender – considering just the males or females in a practice or population
- medically defined problems – physical or mental disease (e.g. heart disease or depression)
- problems identified by communities – access to services, lack of social amenities, fear of crime etc.
- self-defined problems such as pain symptoms or disability.

Therefore the relationship between need, want and demand may be different for different problems.

# Process and definition of HNA

Many methods have been described for undertaking HNA. These are designed to investigate the diverse aspects and perspectives of need and HNA described above. In order to choose the appropriate method and focus on the appropriate population group, it is important to:

- define the purpose of the investigation clearly
- have an understanding of the type and likely results of the HNA (based on previous research and one's experience and common sense)
- have an understanding of what is likely to be involved in subsequent action plans.

Therefore, although there are many different interpretations of what constitutes HNA, HNA should be considered to be much more than just data collection.[73,74] HNA should be regarded as the total process whereby a problem is identified either reactively or from a proactive investigation, investigated, solutions identified to address the problem and action plans devised to implement the solutions.[56] Thus, HNA can be considered to comprise similar elements to the clinical audit cycle and research methodology, namely:

- identification of a problem and formulation of a question to be asked
- choice of an appropriate methodology(s) to answer/obtain information about the problem, including current resources and service provision – as appropriate
- analysis of the information obtained to identify the 'gaps' between current and desired position
- identification of solutions to the issues from the analysis
- development of action plans/strategies to implement the solutions
- implementation of the action plans

- evaluation of the impact of the plans and review of the solutions in the light of this evaluation
- development of further action plans and implementation as necessary.

## Methodologies for HNA: identifying variations and inequalities

Variations and inequalities may be identified in a number of ways – reactively or proactively.

*Reactively*, a health professional may identify a problem during his/her routine practice. This may be through experiencing difficulties in arranging appropriate care for a patient because of waiting times for outpatients, lack of beds for emergency admission, lack of provision of certain treatments and so on. A patient or carer may raise the problem either directly or through a complaints procedure.

*Proactively*, the problem may come to light through analysis of routinely available information on the practice, PCT or hospital trust or from national data. This may be provided by the local public health department or arise from an investigation/'HNA' undertaken by the practice.[75] Routine local authority information may also provide evidence of local health problems.

In addition, HNA may be conducted at a number of levels, depending on the nature of the problem and the population being considered.[76] These particularly include the following.

- *The individual patient/carer level* – interactions at this level are often regarded as being doctor–patient consultations. However, such needs assessment may involve any representative of any profession or organisation that a person with a perceived health need approaches for help, whether the approach was initiated by the patient or the professional. This representative's task is to translate the perceived health need or problem into a healthcare need, as previously defined. This usually takes little account of the wider community interests. The degree to which the person with the problem is involved is a matter of style of the health professional involved.

  Involving people in the decision-making process is more likely to result in a satisfied person who will comply with the treatment, investigations or referral that is mutually agreed.[77,78] Although partly a question of consultation style, patients are becoming more ready to question the 'best judgement' of their physician and are thus involving themselves in the decision-making process.
- *NHS organisational level* – the current trend, as part of the NHS reforms, is to involve users of the services, whether they be patients, relatives or carers.

This is by a process of consumer satisfaction questionnaires produced by hospitals, wards, departments and by general practices. By asking questions about waiting times, courtesy, instructions on getting to the service, food and other process issues, areas needing improvement are identified.

- *Community level* – assessment at this level involves more formal research methodologies in the form of surveys (quantitative and qualitative, rapid appraisal and so on).[79,80]

The sources of information and investigation method(s) chosen should be determined by the purpose of the enquiry. For example, is the exercise aimed at a medically identified need? If so, is it aimed at one particular disease or illness or is it attempting to address all types of illness in the community? Will it be based on patient-defined symptoms or on medical diagnosis? Will the diagnosis be based on medical opinion or supported by objective investigation? Will the HNA be directed towards problems identified by the local community? In which case, they may not be 'medically' definable health problems at all, though will impact on the health of the population, e.g. noise pollution, fear of crime, lack of social amenities or dangerous roads and so on.

The following list gives a flavour of both the sources of further information and the methodologies by which it can be obtained:

- routine information sources (*see* Chapter 1)
- reviews of local services
- rapid appraisal[79,81]
- life-cycle methodology[82]
- narrative-based medicine[83,84]
- HNA in primary care[85–87]
- government plans for the NHS, e.g. *The NHS Plan, Shifting the Balance of Power*[88,89]
- using complaints systems
- using critical incidents
- using quality of life measures[90,91]
- other ways may include setting up systems within primary care and PCTs for front-line workers to pass on problems they identify in their everyday work; these can then be collated and, where difficulties point to a more generalised problem, action plans (strategies) can be developed to tackle them.

Different approaches to applying these techniques are also described. *Epidemiological* enquiry is based on acquisition of knowledge through research. The *corporate* approach involves all interested parties, both professional and lay people. The *comparative* approach involves the comparison of one area with another in terms of need and use of resources.[62,92]

# Health needs assessment: health warning

As we have seen, HNA is much more than just collecting information, and planning services and actions is more than extrapolating directly from the results of the HNA. Therefore, it is important to understand the limitations of the HNA methodologies before jumping to conclusions based on the analysis of the HNA. The following health warnings are worth noting.

- *Quantitative data*: information on incidence and prevalence of the problem is valuable, particularly in HNAs that focus on specific types of disease or disability. However, even if data about incidence and prevalence is available, it is often derived from studies of other populations. Thus, any inference about a local population often comes with wide confidence intervals (*see* Chapter 1). For planning purposes this may not be very helpful as the difference between the upper and lower confidence intervals may represent many hundreds of thousands of pounds or large numbers of personnel, when translated into planning terms.
- *HNA and service use*: there is poor understanding of the relationship between assessed need and use of services. People vary in their use of services. Research has identified a number of barriers that people feel affect their ability to access services.[93,94]
- *HNA and interventions*: once the problem is identified there may not necessarily be agreement about the interventions to be provided. Even with good research evidence there is likely to be inter-professional disagreements and where there is little specific evidence then there is wide scope for argument. Often there is little evidence of effective interventions on which to base a decision, although no evidence does not mean interventions do not work. They may be taken as self-evident or regarded as so routine that a randomised trial would not be possible. These and other related issues are discussed in Chapters 3 and 9.
- *Expectations*: Neither the organisation/personnel involved in the investigation nor the group under investigation should have unrealistic expectations of the outcomes of any HNA, in terms of reconfiguration of services or new developments. The personnel who can authorise such changes need to be involved from the beginning so that everyone is aware of the resources that are likely to be available. In circumstances where this is not the case, there can be a lot of wasted effort which could have been directed to something more useful – there is always too much to do! This not only misdirects resources but generates cynicism which may have a negative effect on future attempts at improving services. There are numerous examples of HNAs that look nice in a report but are gathering dust on a shelf and local communities that have 'been researched to death' but resulted in little tangible benefit.[75]

- *Resources*: Action on the results of an HNA may be contingent on there being resources available to effect any change. Extra resources may not always be necessary and often a reconfiguration of a service within the current resource can lead to great improvements. Nevertheless, many HNAs will identify deficiencies and gaps in the service that do require additional resources. Thus, consideration of how resources may be made available to tackle the results of an HNA needs to be considered before embarking on the HNA, otherwise people become despondent if nothing comes of all their hard work.

The government may decide on the total financial envelope allocated to the NHS but this is influenced by how much they gauge the public are willing to pay in taxes. Budgetary constraints will certainly influence how much can be provided, but should this be the first consideration or should level of need be the driving force for determining the size of the financial envelope?[95,96]

Services can also be funded from other sources: privately, Health Action Zone monies, European funding streams, regeneration budgets and so on. Whether these monies are 'bid' for may be determined by professionals in the local health community and their assessment of need. If a 'bid' is made it may be deemed unsuccessful by a central group – perhaps on the basis of a poorly presented 'bid' or there being too much competition, rather than by the assessment or level of need within that particular community. If the 'bid' is successful, how the money is spent may or may not involve lay people, and even if it does, how representative are they and how should they be selected?

The total budget for a particular locality therefore is variable, over and above the NHS allocation, and only partly based on some estimate of need.

Thus, although there are (and it is intended there should be) links between health needs assessment, commissioning services and resources, these links are not direct or straightforward. The actions to meet gaps in services identified through HNA are expressed in the health strategy for the community – the local health improvement programme (HImP). Through the commissioning process and the Service and Financial Framework (SaFF), priorities are chosen or, rather, as many services as can be afforded within the funding available are purchased. The HImP and SaFF processes are now brought together as the local development plan (LDP). However, other services not selected may be funded through the other streams mentioned or by developing partnerships with pharmaceutical companies, private sources or other funding bodies such as the British Heart Foundation etc.

Issues relating to resource allocation and priority setting are the concern of Section 3.

**Exercise 5.3**

- Describe the different perspectives and dimensions involved in defining *need.*
- Describe a strategy for assessing health needs from the perspective of:
  - a general practice
  - a primary care trust
  - a trust hospital.
- Discuss how these different perspectives may be aligned at a health community (district) level.

# Section 3: Rationing/priority setting/resource allocation

Decisions concerning allocation of resources occur at all levels of the NHS. The government determines the overall financial allocation to all the public services – education, environment, health and so on. However, the basis on which the level of funding is determined is unclear. This money is then cascaded down the system to front-line services. The routes by which this occurs have changed over the years and are currently undergoing further change with a more direct line from government to the commissioners, i.e. PCTs.

A number of methodologies have been tried to ensure distribution of resources bears some relationship to level of need.[97–102] Such formulas aim to redress the historical situation whereby London and the more affluent South of the country receive proportionately more funding than the more deprived areas of the North. This has not been entirely successful.[102] However, this is not the only level at which decisions about resource allocation are made. Individual health professionals, their unions and professional bodies and the organisations for which they work make judgements and recommendations about time allocation for patients and for other duties. Hospitals and PCTs decide how many staff and services they can provide within the total funding envelope available to the local health community. The most visible consequences of these decisions are the waiting times patients endure to see their GP or hospital consultant or receive an operation and the variability in service provision between local health communities* and within local hospital trusts. This is no better illustrated than in the so-called concept of 'treatment by postcode'. This occurs where health communities make different commissioning decisions, particularly in respect of the provision of new drugs. Thus, depending in which local health community one lives, one may or may not receive a particular therapy.[103]

## Terminology

The words used are important in describing the fact that decisions are clearly being made resulting in limitations of access to healthcare provision. To some extent it depends on the impression the particular user wishes to create. *Rationing* is very emotive and creates the impression that there are 'insufficient

---

* In this context, the health community refers to what was the health authority, but now is one or several PCT(s) – organisations that are making decisions for populations served by a number of general practices. Such populations may cover part, one or a number of local authority areas.

resources' to go round. If this is the case, it clearly lies at the government's door. Not unnaturally, the government is not happy to accept this conclusion as it may have a negative effect on voters. They therefore use the word *priority*, and explicitly give the responsibility to local health communities. This implies that some sort of 'pseudo-scientific' process is undertaken by 'local experts' armed with sufficient wisdom and knowledge, resulting in a fair and affordable basket of services to meet the needs of the local population. This does not really happen in practice – how does the importance and benefit of total hip replacement compare to dietary advice for obese children? Notwithstanding the inherent difficulty of such a question, the government 'must-be-dones' of waiting list numbers etc. also distort the flexibility to make local decisions. Given the local funding envelope, services not chosen for funding are then deemed not to be a priority. This gives the wrong messages to those needing such services.

What tends to happen in practice is that commissioning is guided by historical precedent and government targets. Resources are then spread as widely as possible to provide as many different services as can be afforded, given the other priority of balancing the books. *Resource allocation* is an accurate description of what is taking place but of course gives no indication of how this occurs. Lack of adequate provision can then be 'blamed' on poor decision making rather than an absolute lack of resources. Currently, the government is taking a lead on directing resources, but without acknowledging the rationing dimension. This is through the use of special funds, e.g. the Modernisation Fund, and by 'earmarking' funds, within the baseline allocations, for certain conditions, and also by issuing National Service Frameworks which stipulate types of service to be provided.

It is generally accepted that not every treatment can be provided for every patient as and when they require it.[104,105] This is based on the assumption that the health needs or demands of the population outstrip not only current resources but almost any amount of increased future resource the government may choose to throw at the NHS. Although this proposition is not universally accepted, some mechanism of limiting expenditure on the NHS is assumed to be necessary.[106,107] The crux of the matter is how best to balance the demand and supply sides of the equation in a way that is seen to be fair and provides a reasonable and effective service.

Funding systems other than solely by government have been discussed.[108,109] Although it is essential to review the most effective and efficient ways of funding health, one gets the impression that the underlying belief for seeking alternatives to funding from taxation is to circumvent the need to engage in a rationing debate. The supplementary role of the private sector and other funding streams also needs consideration. Other health systems are having similar debates and different solutions have been advocated and tried.[110–115]

However, as Klein argues, there is no technical fix to the dilemma of rationing.[116] He suggests that what is necessary is an open and honest review of the decision-making processes from government, the Department of Health and down to individual clinicians. This will make for better decision making and more understanding from the public of the constraints the system is under.

Thus, the following are the main points to consider.

- At what level should rationing decisions be made – national or local level or a combination of the two?[110,117–118]
- Who should be involved in the decision-making process and how – professionals, the public?[119–120]
- Establishing an open and inclusive process, nationally and locally, i.e. should some representative group be constituted to consider these issues?
- Which principles should be the basis of an ethical framework and considerations of vertical and horizontal equity (i.e. rationing within specific services, e.g. orthopaedics, and between services, e.g. orthopaedics and ophthalmology)?[121–128]
- Which issues should be considered – individual cases, a basket of services decided locally, all services but with limitations on access, introduction of new technologies and service developments within the health community, a basket of services to be decided nationally?[129–131]

## Consequences of rationing decisions

At a national level, rationing healthcare is seen as a vote loser and hence all governments have shied away from really confronting the reality of scarce resources and talking openly of limiting services. The responsibility of deciding what to do with the resources allocated is left to local health communities. This very often means that individual clinicians make rationing decisions within consultations with individual patients. Often, such decisions are not recognised as such and may be made on the grounds of clinical appropriateness. However, funding pressures within the system may have an undue effect, often subconsciously, on clinicians as they make these decisions. This is because clinical judgement is not a precise scientific process and all sorts of factors play a part in the final outcome.

This is an inappropriate position for clinicians to be in. If a group, broadly representative of the local community, has agreed criteria in another forum, then it is reasonable for clinicians to be the ones who apply them in individual situations. However, in this instance the responsibility is shared for not making certain treatments available. This is important as one of the knock-on effects of rationing and limiting access to particular services is the risk of complaint and litigation from members of the community who are denied these treatments.

Thus, to limit the risk of formal complaint and judicial review, it is necessary to demonstrate that the decision-making process is as fair and open as possible.[132–133] Apart from the time and stress caused by complaints, the financial burden on the NHS is such that it diverts considerable resources away from patient services. It is therefore good risk management to ensure a robust decision-making process is in place.

# Case studies

The following case studies are used to explore different dimensions of resource allocation. The first uses beta interferon to highlight the dilemmas associated with introducing new technologies into the NHS. The second highlights the specific situation in which a particular patient requests his/her particular doctor to provide access to a treatment not provided routinely by the health community. The third presents a number of competing requests for funding and illustrates the factors to be considered in choosing between them.

---

**Case study 1**

**So few, so much and so little**

Beta interferon was in use in a number of countries before being given a licence for use in the UK in 1996. The licence was issued for use in a specific group of patients – relapsing/remitting type of multiple sclerosis (MS). The government-issued guidance, Executive Letter EL(95)97, indicated the parameters for use. It included reference to EL(94)72 concerning the introduction of new drugs into the NHS and included the advice from the Standing Medical Advisory Committee (SMAC guidance) on the use of beta interferon. The British Society of Neurologists also issued guidance in 1999. A further piece of guidance, Health Service Circular (HSC) 1999/999, was issued indicating that further guidance would be issued and the National Institute for Clinical Excellence (NICE) would be asked to make recommendations for using beta interferon.

These pieces of guidance have provided the framework for health communities to make their decision as to whether they will provide therapy or not. Although the guidance is based on research evidence, a number of health communities have determined that the cost benefit of this treatment is too high and have chosen not to provide treatment. Other health communities have taken the opposite view or at least have chosen to follow government guidance about not imposing 'blanket bans' and are providing treatment pending deliberations by NICE.

---

**Case study 2**

**Please doctor, can I have ...?**

Mrs Parkinson believes she is suffering from multiple allergies. She feels she has tried everything the local health service can offer but is no better. She has talked with friends and has found on the Internet the 'Cure It All' private clinic. She arranges an assessment. The medical director of the clinic tells her that she requires further tests, a course of desensitisation and tablets to replace several mineral deficiencies. She takes the results of the assessment to her GP and requests treatment on the NHS. The GP contacts the PCT for advice.

**Exercise 5.4**

- What factors should be taken into account in determining the usefulness of a particular therapy or service?
- What additional factors/principles should be considered in deciding whether or not to provide a particular therapy or service?
- Who could make such decisions? What options are there?
- How should such decisions be made?

**Case study 3**

**Damned if you do and ...**

1   The health community require to increase their cardiac revascularisation rates by 10% per annum to meet the requirements of the National Service Framework by 2010. This means an annual increase in investment of £200 000. In addition, the tertiary centre will require more investment to provide the capacity to meet this activity level.
2   The local orthopaedic review has determined that two more surgeons are required if they are to meet their waiting-time targets and increase their joint replacement rates to the national average. This will cost approximately £200 000, plus the costs of the increased activity.
3   Eight practices each need two full-time practice nurses to provide the full range of services required by the PCT. This will cost about £200 000.

The health community has identified about £200 000 of development monies for the coming year. What should be funded?

Although this example appears contrived, the reality of the commissioning process throws up the need for choices in this stark way. The following questions draw out the factors that have to be taken into account and also give an opportunity to consider the process by which these choices can be made and communicated to both the health community and the population.

---

**Exercise 5.5**

- What information is required to inform this situation?
- Is it all of one and nothing of the others?
- How can the decisions be communicated to those concerned?
- What may be the consequences of decisions made?

---

# Comments and approaches to the exercises

The intention of this section is not to provide all the answers (in most cases, there are no right answers), but to provide pointers to the questions, areas or approaches one might take to direct further thinking about the issues. Some of the questions refer directly to the text or associated references and therefore no further comment is made.

## Exercise 5.1

- **List the factors that may be involved in the development of variation in people's experience of health and health services.**

They will include:

- access to services
- level of income
- availability of transport
- educational attainment
- knowledge
- upbringing
- housing conditions and local environment
- service provision and availability
- clinical decision making and use of evidence-based medicine, guidelines and protocols by local health services
- total resource allocation available locally
- pressure from lobby groups
- government priorities – 'must-be-dones'
- historical contracting arrangements, as opposed to commissioning based on health needs of the whole community, and quality of local decision-making processes
- lifestyle behaviours – exercise, smoking, diet, alcohol intake.

- **Which of these could be classed as inequitable?**

What factors influence each of those examples in the list above in determining whether the effect is inequitable?

- What factors affect what you eat?
- Are these dependent on personal choice or institutionalised social factors, i.e. do you know what is healthy?
- Can you afford to choose to eat healthy food?
- Can you cook it?
- Do you have access to it – can you get to an out-of-town supermarket or is the local shop your only option?

- **What theories have been proposed to explain variations in health?**

A number of suggestions have been put forward to explain these differences. These are:

- the artefact thesis
- the behavioural thesis
- the selection thesis
- the material thesis.

See the following further reading.

- Blane D, Davey-Smith G and Bartley M (1990) Social class differences in years of potential life lost: size, trends and principal causes. *BMJ*. **301**: 429–32.
- Townsend P and Davidson N (1982) *Inequalities in Health: The Black Report*. Penguin, London.

## Exercise 5.2

- **Using your own knowledge and local health statistics and information (*see* Chapter 1), identify specific examples of variations in health and in service provision in your area.**

For example:

- Is the mortality rate for lung cancer or coronary heart disease (CHD) the same in all wards of the local authority?
- Are consultation rates of referral rates the same in all GP practices?

- **Apply the two *key* questions to your chosen example *or* to an example of differences in:**
  - **mortality or morbidity**
  - **clinical decision making**
  - **access to healthcare/'postcode' services (*see* Section 3).**

- Consider the causation of the problem, i.e. if smoking is the main cause of lung cancer, what factors influence people's smoking habits? What interventions affect people's smoking habits?
- What factors affect a person's decision to consult his/her doctor? Can these be influenced nationally or locally? What actions can be taken which may affect the different dimensions involved?
- What factors influence a clinician's decision to refer for specialist advice? Consider factors affecting the patient, the doctor, the potential condition (diagnosis, tests, treatment), potential prognosis, effect of uncertainty, costs, geographical location of services.

- **Choose one of the identified inequalities and devise an action plan or strategy to tackle the issue, using the framework set out in Chapter 6.**

- What interventions affect people's smoking habits?
- Which people or organisations should be involved in planning and implementing the strategy? Think of partnerships required to increase the likelihood of developing a comprehensive strategy and encouraging ownership among those expected to resource it and implement it (*see* Chapter 10).

## Exercise 5.3

- **Describe the different perspectives and dimensions involved in defining *need*.**
- **Describe a strategy for assessing health needs from the perspective of:**
  - **a general practice**
  - **a primary care trust**
  - **a trust hospital.**

- Does the approach differ if approached from the perspective of a specific disease, an identified problem or a 'general' HNA?
- Consider the populations involved.
- What are the implications of the HNA – funding, possible interventions, personnel?

- **Discuss how these different perspectives may be aligned at a health community (district level).**

- List the advantages in different organisations carrying out their own HNAs.
- List the disadvantages in different organisations carrying out their own HNAs.
- How might these disadvantages be overcome?
- What benefits are there from joint working? (*See* Chapters 4 and 7.)

## Exercise 5.4

- **What factors should be taken into account in determining the usefulness of a particular therapy or service?**

Consider issues of:

- efficacy and effectiveness of the intervention
- safety and side effects
- patient participation in the decision – not all patients want all treatments
- contraindications
- the place of the new intervention in the whole of the services provided for that condition.

- **What additional factors/principles should be considered in deciding whether or not to provide a particular therapy or service?**

Consider issues relating to:

- cost effectiveness and cost benefits
- fairness
- equity
- opportunity costs – money spent on one service cannot be spent on another, i.e. money can only be spent once. Therefore what services will not be provided if the money is spent in a particular way?

- **Who could make such decisions? What options are there?**

- Consider the advantages and disadvantages of having either an individual or a multidisciplinary group responsible for deciding these issues.
- What disciplines might be represented on a multidisciplinary group and why?
- What role may such a multidisciplinary group play? Consider:
  - decisions on behalf of individual patients, both routinely and in emergencies where a decision is required quickly[133]
  - decisions relating to the introduction of new technologies and interventions
  - decisions encompassing the whole of local service provision.

- **How should such decisions be made?**

Devise a practical 'organisational' structure that would allow decisions to be taken, involve appropriate people, take note of appropriate information, provide for decisions to be disseminated appropriately and recognise the need for an appeals process. (*See* Figure 5.1.)

## Exercise 5.5

- **What information is required to inform this situation and support the decision-making process?**
- **Is it all of one and nothing of the others?**

- If possible, discuss the situation with colleagues involved in commissioning services.
- In practice, there may be a number of ways in which this dilemma may be approached. However, it is unlikely that all three requests can be completely satisfied. Potential options include the following.
  - There may be ways of deferring the commencement of some of the options until later in the year and therefore only incurring part-year costs. Clearly the full-year effect will then need to be picked up the following year.

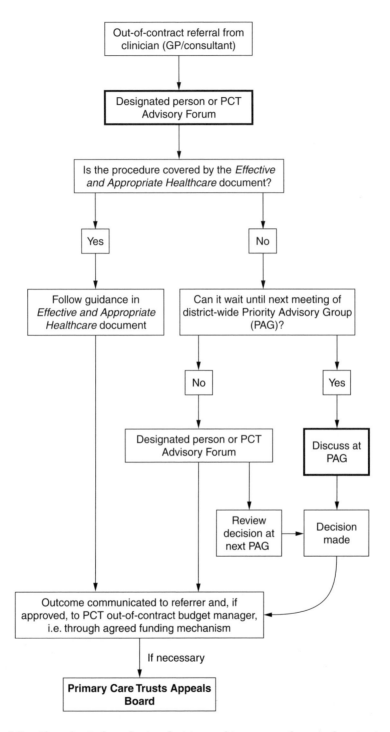

**Figure 5.1:** Flow chart of purchasing decision-making process for out-of-contract procedures.

- It may be possible to use other sources of funding – New Opportunities Fund, HAZ funding, European money, private finance and so on.
- 'Slippage' money may be available, i.e. money allocated for other purposes which has not been spent as the projects have been delayed and will therefore not require all their financial allocations in that year.

- **How can the decisions be communicated to those concerned?**

- Devise a communications strategy to include all those who should be informed of the decisions of such a group.
- Who needs to know?
- What consultation process is required for ratifying the decisions?

- **What may be the consequences of decisions made?**

Consider this question from different perspectives.

- The patient perspective – how do patients react if they are denied access to treatment?
- The healthcare community perspective – how should disagreements be resolved?
- How can the potential for being open to being taken to judicial review be addressed?

# References

1 Townsend P and Davidson N (1982) *Inequalities in Health: The Black Report*. Penguin, London.

2 Wilkinson R (1992) Income distribution and life expectancy. *BMJ*. **304**: 165–8.

3 Blane D, Davey-Smith G and Bartley M (1990) Social class differences in years of potential life lost: size, trends and principal causes. *BMJ*. **301**: 429–32.

4 Haynes R (1991) Inequalities in health and health service use: evidence from the General Household Survey. *Social Science and Medicine*. **33**(4): 361–8.

5 Blaxter M (1990) *Health and Lifestyles*. Tavistock/Routledge, London.

6 Marmot M and Theorell T (1988) Social class and cardiovascular disease: the contribution of work. *International Journal of Health Services*. **18**(4): 659–74.

7 Goldblatt P (ed.) (1990) *Longitudinal Study: mortality and social organisation 1971–1981*. OPCS series LS No. 6. HMSO, London.

8 Whitehead M (1992) *The Health Divide*. Penguin, London.

9 Drever F and Bunting J (1997) Patterns and trends in male mortality. In: F Drever and M Whitehead (eds) *Health Inequalities: decennial supplement*. DS series No.15. The Stationery Office, London.

10 Harding S, Bethune A, Maxwell R and Brown J (1997) Mortality trends using the longitudinal study. In: F Drever and M Whitehead (eds) *Health Inequalities: decennial supplement*. DS series No.15. The Stationery Office, London.

11  Hattersly L (1997) Expectation of life by social class. In: F Drever and M Whitehead (eds) *Health Inequalities: decennial supplement*. The Stationery Office, London.

12  Dahlgren G and Whitehead M (1991) *Policies and Strategies to Promote Social Equity in Health*. Institute for Future Studies, Stockholm (Mimeo).

13  World Bank (1993) *World Development Report 1993: investing in health*. Oxford University Press, New York.

14  Illsley R and Baker D (1997) *Inequalities in Health: adapting the theory to fit the facts*. University of Bath, Centre for the Analysis of Social Policy, Bath.

15  Department of Health (1998) *Independent Inquiry into Inequalities in Health Report (The Acheson Report)*. DoH, London.

16  Barker D (1998) *Mothers, Babies and Health in Later Life*. Churchill Livingstone, Edinburgh.

17  Montgomery S and Schoon I (1997) Health and health behaviour. In: J Bynner, E Ferri and P Shepherd (eds) *Twentysomething in the 1990s: getting on, getting by, getting nowhere*. Ashgate, Aldershot.

18  Bynner J and Parsons S (1997) *It Doesn't Get Any Better: the impact of poor basic skills on the lives of 37 year olds*. The Basic Skills Agency, London.

19  Burridge R and Ormandy D (eds) (1993) *Unhealthy Housing: research, remedies and reform*. E and FN Spon, London.

20  Arblaster L and Hawtin M (1993) *Health, Housing and Social Policy*. Socialist Health Association, London.

21  Platt S, Martin C, Hunt S and Lewis C (1989) Damp housing, mould growth and symptomatic health state. *BMJ*. **298**: 1673–8.

22  Strachan D (1988) Damp housing and childhood asthma: validation of reporting of symptoms. *BMJ*. **297**: 1223–6.

23  Best R (1994) The Duke of Edinburgh's Inquiry into British Housing: three years on. In: Ford J and Wilcox S (eds) *Housing Finance Review 1994/5*. Joseph Rowntree Foundation, York.

24  Ravelli A, van der Meulen J, Michels R *et al*. (1998) Glucose tolerance in adults after prenatal exposure to the Dutch famine. *Lancet*. **351**: 173–7.

25  Clark P, Allen C, Law C, Shiell A, Godfrey K and Barker D (1998) Weight gain in pregnancy, triceps skinfold thickness and blood pressure in the offspring. *Obstetrics and Gynecology*. **91**: 103–7.

26  Godfrey K, Forrester T, Barker D *et al*. (1994) Maternal nutritional status in pregnancy and blood pressure in childhood. *British Journal of Obstetrics and Gynaecology*. **101**: 398–403.

27  Forsen T, Eriksson J, Tuomilehto J, Teramo K, Osmond C and Barker D (1997) Mother's weight in pregnancy and coronary heart disease in a cohort of Finnish men: follow-up study. *BMJ*. **315**: 837–40.

28  Campbell D, Hall M, Barker D, Cross J, Shiell A and Godfrey K (1996) Diet in pregnancy and the offspring's blood pressure 40 years later. *British Journal of Obstetrics and Gynaecology*. **103**: 273–80.

29  James W, Nelson M, Ralph A and Leather S (1997) The contribution of nutrition to inequalities in health. *BMJ*. **314**: 1545–9.

30  Morris JN (1994) Exercise in the prevention of coronary heart disease: today's best buy in public health. *Medicine and Science in Sports and Exercise*. **26**: 807–14.

31 Wannamathee G, Shaper AG and Walker M (1998) Changes in physical activity, mortality and incidence of coronary heart disease in older men. *Lancet*. **352**: 1603–8.

32 US Surgeon General (1996) *Physical Activity and Health. A report of the Surgeon General*. US Department of Health and Human Services, Washington, DC.

33 Benzeval M, Judge K and Smaje C (1995) Beyond class, race and ethnicity: deprivation and health in Britain. *Health Services Research*. Special issue. **30**(1).

34 Dobson B, Beardsworth A, Keil T and Walker R (1994) *Diet, Choice and Poverty: social, cultural and nutritional aspects of food consumption among low income families*. Loughborough University of Technology, Centre for Research in Social Policy, Loughborough.

35 Dowler E and Calvert C (1995) *Nutrition and Diet in Lone-parent Families in London*. Family Policy Studies Centre, London.

36 Lobstein T (1991) *The Nutrition of Women on Low Income*. Food Commission, London.

37 Markus T (1993) Cold, condensation and housing poverty. In: R Burridge and D Ormandy (eds) *Unhealthy Housing: research, remedies and reform*. E and FN Spon, London.

38 Savage A (1988) *Warmth in Winter: evaluation of an information pack for elderly people*. University of Wales College of Medicine Research Team for the Care of the Elderly, Cardiff.

39 Drever F and Whitehead M (eds) (1997) *Health Inequalities: decennial supplement*. DS series No. 15. The Stationery Office, London.

40 McCormick A, Flemming D and Charlton J (1995) *Morbidity Statistics from General Practice: fourth national study: 1991–1992*. A study carried out by the Royal College of General Practitioners, the Office of Population Censuses and Surveys of the Department of Health. OPCS series MB5 No. 3. HMSO, London.

41 Lawless P, Martin R and Hardy S (1998) *Unemployment and Social Exclusion: landscapes of labour inequality*. Jessica Kingsley Publishers, London.

42 Nickell S and Bell B (1995) The collapse in demand for the unskilled and unemployment across the OECD. *Oxford Review of Economic Policy: unemployment*. **11**: 40–62.

43 Payne J and Payne C (1994) Trends in job loss and recruitment in Britain 1979–1991. In: M White (ed.) *Unemployment and Public Policy in a Changing Labour Market*. Policy Studies Institute, London.

44 Bartley M (1994) Unemployment and health: understanding the relationship. *Journal of Epidemiology and Community Health*. **48**: 333–7.

45 Shortt S (1996) Is unemployment pathogenic? A review of current concepts with lessons for policy planners. *International Journal of Health Services*. **26**: 569–89.

46 Bethune A (1997) Unemployment and mortality. In: F Drever and M Whitehead (eds) *Health Inequalities: decennial supplement*. DS series No.15. The Stationery Office, London.

47 Moser K, Goldblatt P, Fox J and Jones D (1990) Unemployment and mortality. In: P Goldblatt (ed.) *Longitudinal Study 1971–1981: mortality and social organisation*. HMSO, London.

48 Green G, Grimsley M, Soukas A, Prescott M, Jowitt T and Linacre R (2000) *Social Capital, Health and Economy in South Yorkshire Coalfield Communities*. Centre for Regional Economic and Social Research, Sheffield Hallam University, Sheffield.

49 Campbell C, Wood R and Kelly M (1999) *Social Capital and Health*. Health Education Authority, London.

50 Department of Health Committee on the Medical Effects of Air Pollutants (1998) *Quantification of the Effects of Air Pollution on Health in the United Kingdom*. The Stationery Office, London.

51 Benzeval M, Judge K and Whitehead M (eds) (1995) *Tackling Inequalities in Health: an agenda for action*. King's Fund, London.

52 Department of Health (1995) *Variations in Health. What can the Department of Health and the NHS do?* DoH, London.

53 Eachus J, Chan P, Pearson N, Propper C and Davey Smith G (1999) An additional dimension to health inequalities: disease severity and socioeconomic position. *Journal of Epidemiology and Community Health.* **53**(10): 603–11.

54 Department of Health (1994) *On the State of the Public Health. The Annual Report of the Chief Medical Officer of Health*. HMSO, London.

55 Department of Health (2001) *Tackling Health Inequalities – consultation on a plan for delivery*. DoH, London.

56 Wright J, Williams R and Wilkinson JR (1998) Development and importance of health needs assessment. *BMJ.* **316**: 1310–13.

57 Harrison A, Dixon J, New B and Judge K (1997) Funding the NHS. Can the NHS cope in future? *BMJ.* **314**: 139–42.

58 Ham C (1993) Priority setting in the NHS: reports from six districts. *BMJ.* **307**: 435–8.

59 Stronks K, Strijbis A-M, Wendte JF and Gunning-Schepers LJ (1997) Who should decide? Qualitative analysis of panel data from public, patients, healthcare professionals and insurers on priorities in health care. *BMJ.* **315**: 92–6.

60 Heginbotham C (1993) Health care priority setting: a survey of doctors, managers and the general public. In: *Rationing in Action*. BMJ Publishing Group, London.

61 Bradshaw JR (1972) A taxonomy of social need. In: G McLachlan (ed.) *Problems and Progress in Medical Care: essays on current research*. 7th series. Oxford University Press, Oxford.

62 Stevens A and Raftery J (Vol. 1 1994, Vol. 2 1997) *Health Care Needs Assessment: the epidemiology based needs assessment reviews*. Radcliffe Medical Press, Oxford.

63 Dolan P (2001) Utilitarianism and the measurement and aggregation of quality-adjusted life years. *Health Care Analysis.* **9**(1): 65–76.

64 Raisch DW (2000) Understanding quality-adjusted life years and their application to pharmacoeconomic research. *Annals of Pharmacotherapy.* **34**(7–8): 906–14.

65 Brazier J, Deverill M and Green C (1999) A review of the use of health status measures in economic evaluation. *Journal of Health Services and Research Policy.* **4**(3): 174–84.

66 Deverill M, Brazier J, Green C and Booth A (1998) The use of QALY and non-QALY measures of health-related quality of life. Assessing the state of the art. *Pharmacoeconomics.* **13**(4): 411–20.

67 Arnesen T and Nord E (1999) The value of DALY life: problems with ethics and validity of disability adjusted life years. *BMJ.* **319**: 1423–5.

68 Arnesen T and Nord E (2000) The value of DALY life: problems with ethics and validity of disability adjusted life years. *Leprosy Review.* **71**(2): 123–7.

69 Rawles J (1989) Castigating QALYs. *Journal of Medical Ethics.* **15**: 143.

70 Bradshaw JR (1994) The conceptualisation and measurement of need. A social policy perspective. In: J Popay and G Williams (eds) *Researching the People's Health*. Routledge, London.

71 Maslow A (1954) *Motivation and Personality.* Harper and Row, London.

72 Hannay DR (1979) *The Symptom Iceberg: a study of community health.* Routledge, London.

73 Robinson J and Elkan R (1996) *Health Needs Assessment, Theory and Practice.* Churchill Livingstone, London.

74 Gillam S and Murray S (1996) *Needs Assessment in General Practice.* Occasional Paper 73. Royal College of General Practitioners, London.

75 Williams G and Popay J (1994) Dilemmas and opportunities for social scientists. In: J Popay and G Williams (eds) *Researching the People's Health.* Routledge, London.

76 Wilkinson JR and Murray SA (1998) Assessment in primary care: practical issues and possible approaches. *BMJ.* **316**: 1524–8.

77 Little P, Everitt H, Williamson I, Warner G, Moore M, Gould C *et al.* (2001) Preferences of patients for patient centred approach to consultation in primary care: observational study. *BMJ.* **322**: 468–72.

78 Skelton JR (2001) Patients' preferences for patient centred approach to consultation. What is patient centredness? *BMJ.* **322**: 1544.

79 Ong BN and Humphris G (1994) Prioritising needs with communities. Rapid Appraisal methodologies in health. In: J Popay and G Williams (eds) *Researching the People's Health.* Routledge, London.

80 Ong BN, Humphris G, Annett H and Rifkin S (1991) Rapid Appraisal in an urban setting: an example from the developed world. *Social Science and Medicine.* **32**(8): 909–15.

81 Murray S (1999) Experiences with 'rapid appraisal' in primary care: involving the public in assessing health needs, orientating staff and educating students. *BMJ.* **318**: 440–4.

82 Pickin C and St Leger S (1993) *Assessing Health Needs Using the Life Cycle Framework.* Open University Press, Buckingham.

83 Elwyn G and Gwyn R (1999) Narrative based medicine: stories we hear and stories we tell: analysing talk in clinical practice. *BMJ.* **318**: 186–8.

84 Greenhalgh T and Hurwitz B (1999) Narrative based medicine: why study narrative? *BMJ.* **318**: 48–50.

85 Ruta DA, Duffy MC, Farquharson A, Young AM, Gilmour FB and McElduff SP (1997) Determining priorities for change in primary care: the value of practice-based needs assessment. *British Journal of General Practice.* **47**: 353–7.

86 Hooper J and Longworth P (1997) *Health Needs Assessment in Primary Care: a workbook for primary health care teams.* Calderdale and Kirklees Health Authority, Wakefield.

87 Gillam S, Plampling D, McClennan J, Harries J and Epstein L (1994) *Community Orientated Primary Care.* King's Fund, London.

88 Department of Health (2001) *NHS Plan: a plan for investment, a plan for reform.* DoH, London.

89 Department of Health (2001) *Shifting the Balance of Power Within the NHS: securing delivery.* DoH, London.

90 Bowling A (1991) Health care research methods. Part 2. *Nursing Standard.* **5**(49): 33–5.

91 Bowling A (1991) Health care research methods. Part 1. *Nursing Standard.* **5**(48): 34–7.

92 National Health Service Management Executive (1991) *Assessing Health Care Needs.* Department of Health, London.

93  Tod AM, Read C, Lacey A and Abbot J (2001) Barriers to uptake of services for coronary heart disease: a qualitative study. *BMJ*. **323**: 1–6.

94  Gardner K and Chapple A (1999) Barriers to referral in patients with angina: qualitative study. *BMJ*. **319**: 418–22.

95  Sheldon TA (1997) Formula fever: allocating resources in the NHS. *BMJ*. **315**: 964.

96  Harrison A and Dixon J (2000) *The NHS. Facing the future*. King's Fund, London.

97  Department of Health and Social Security (1976) *Sharing Resources for Health in England* (report of the Resource Allocation Working Party – RAWP). DHSS, London.

98  Department of Health (1989) *Funding and Contracts for Health Services*. Working paper 2. HMSO, London.

99  Sheldon TA, Davey Smith G and Bevan G (1993) Weighting in the dark: resource allocation in the new NHS. *BMJ*. **306**: 835–9.

100  Sheldon TA (1997) Formula fever: allocating resources in the NHS. *BMJ*. **315**: 964.

101  NAHAT (National Association of Health Authorities and Trusts) (1996) *Allocation of resources to the NHS. Briefing 103*. Birmingham Research Park, Birmingham.

102  Peacock S and Smith P (1995) *The Resource Allocation Consequences of the New NHS Needs Formula*. Centre for Health Economics, University of York, York.

103  Redmayne S and Klein R (1993) Rationing in practice: the case of *in vitro* fertilisation. *BMJ*. **306**: 1521.

104  Owen D (1976) In sickness and in health: the politics of medicine. Quoted by: D Black (1991) Paying for health. *Journal of Medical Ethics*. **17**: 117.

105  Sheldon TA and Maynard A (1993) Is rationing inevitable? In: *Rationing in Action*. BMJ Publishing Group, London.

106  Harris T (1993) Consulting the public. In: *Rationing in Action*. BMJ Publishing Group, London.

107  Light DW (1997) The real ethics of rationing. *BMJ*. **314**: 296–8.

108  Harrison A, Dixon J, New B and Judge K (1997) Funding the NHS: is the NHS sustainable? *BMJ*. **314**: 296–8.

109  Harrison A and Dixon J (2000) *The NHS. Facing the future*. King's Fund, London.

110  Oregon Health Services Commission (1991) *Prioritisation of Health Services*. Oregon Health Commission, Salem.

111  Ham C (1998) Retracing the Oregon Trail: the experience of rationing and the Oregon Health Plan. *BMJ*. **316**: 1965–9.

112  Hadorn DC and Holmes AC (1997) The New Zealand priority criteria project. Part 1: overview. *BMJ*. **314**: 131–4.

113  Chinitz D, Shalev C, Galai N and Israeli A (1998) Israel's basic basket of health services: the importance of being explicitly implicit. *BMJ*. **317**: 1005–7.

114  Ministry for Health Welfare and Cultural Affairs (Netherlands) (1992) *Choices in Health Care*. Rijswijk.

115  Ministry for Health and Social Affairs (1995) *No Easy Choices – the difficult priorities on health care*. Stockholm. [The Royal Ministry of Heath and Social Welfare (1987) *Retningdlinjer for prioritering innen Norsk helesetjeneste*. NOU, Oslo.]

116 Klein R (1993) Dimensions of rationing: who should do what? In: *Rationing in Action*. BMJ Publishing Group, London.

117 Lenaghan J (1997) Central Government should have a greater role in rationing decisions. The case for. *BMJ*. **314**: 967–70.

118 Harrison S (1997) Central Government should have a greater role in rationing decisions. The case against. *BMJ*. **314**: 970–3.

119 Stronks K, Strijbis A-M, Wendte JF and Gunning-Schepers LJ (1997) Who should decide? Qualitative analysis of panel data from public, patients, health care professionals and insurers on priorities in health care. *BMJ*. **315**: 92–6.

120 Hope T, Hicks N, Reynolds DJM, Crisp R and Griffiths S (1998) Rationing and the health authority. *BMJ*. **317**: 1067–9.

121 Doyal L (1995) Needs, rights and equity: moral quality in healthcare rationing. *Quality in Health Care*. **4**: 273–83.

122 Culyer AJ (1997) Maximising the health of the whole community. *BMJ*. **314**: 667–9.

123 Williams A (1997) Rationing health care by age. The case for. *BMJ*. **314**: 820–2.

124 Grimley Evans J (1997) Rationing health care by age. The case against. *BMJ*. **314**: 822–5.

125 Doyal L (1997) Rationing within the NHS should be explicit. The case for. *BMJ*. **314**: 1114–18.

126 Coast J (1997) Rationing within the NHS should be explicit. The case against. *BMJ*. **314**: 1118–22.

127 Gillon R (1985) Justice and allocation of medical resources. *BMJ*. **291**: 266.

128 Chadwick R (1993) Justice in priority setting. In: *Rationing in Action*. BMJ Publishing Group, London.

129 New B (1997) Defining a package of healthcare services the NHS is responsible for. The case for. *BMJ*. **314**: 503–5.

130 Klein R (1997) Defining a package of healthcare services the NHS is responsible for. The case against. *BMJ*. **314**: 506–9.

131 *R* v *North Derbyshire Health Authority*, ex parte Fisher (1997) **38** BMLR 76.

132 *R* v *Central Birmingham Health Authority*, ex parte Walker (1987) **3** BMLR 32.

133 *R* v *Cambridge Health Authority*, ex parte Child B (1995) **6** *Med LR* 250.

# Further reading

- Benzeval M, Judge K and Whitehead M (eds) (1995) *Tackling Inequalities in Health: an agenda for action*. King's Fund, London.
- Black D (1990) The Black Report. In: P Townsend and N Davidson (eds) *Inequalities in Health*. Penguin Books, London.
- Blaxter M (1990) *Health and Lifestyles*. Tavistock/Routledge, London.
- Bradshaw JS (1972) A taxonomy of social need. In: G McLachlan (ed.) *Problems and Progress in Medical Care: essays on current research*. 7th series. Oxford University Press, Oxford.

- British Medical Association (1942) *Draft Interim Report of the Medical Planning Commission.* BMA, London.
- Butler J (1999) *The Ethics of Health Care Rationing: principles and practices.* Cassell, London.
- Cormack D (1989) *Peacing Together.* Monarch Publishing, Eastbourne.
- Coulter A and Ham C (eds) (2000) *The Global Challenge of Health Care Rationing.* State of Health series. Open University Press, Buckingham.
- Downie RS, Fyfe C and Tannahill A (1990) *Health Promotion: models and values.* Oxford University Press, Oxford.
- Doyle L (1979) *The Political Economy of Health.* Pluto Press, London.
- Friere P (1970) *Pedagogy of the Opressed.* Seabury Press, New York.
- Friere P (1973) *Education for Critical Consciousness.* Seabury Press, New York.
- Gough I (1978) Theories of the welfare state: a critique. *International Journal of Health Services.* **8**(1).
- Griffiths S and Hunter DJ (eds) (1999) *Perspectives in Public Health.* Radcliffe Medical Press, Oxford.
- Ham C (1992) *Health Policy in Britain. The politics and organisation of the National Health Service.* Macmillan Press Limited, Basingstoke.
- Ham C and McIver S (2000) *Contested Decisions: priority setting in the NHS. Policy dilemmas.* King's Fund, London.
- Hannay DR (1979) *The Symptom Iceberg: a study of community health.* Routledge, London.
- Harrison A and Dixon J (2000) *The NHS. Facing the future.* King's Fund, London.
- Lalonde M (1974) *A New Perspective on the Health of Canadians.* Government of Canada, Ottowa.
- Levitt R and Wall A (1984) *Background to Today's National Health Service. The re-organised National Health Service.* Chapman and Hall, London.
- Maslow A (1954) *Motivation and Personality.* Harper and Row, London.
- Mason JK and McCall Smith RA (1994) *Law and Medical Ethics.* Butterworths, London.
- Navarro V (1986) *Medicine Under Capitalism. Crisis in health and medicine. A social critique.* Tavistock, London.
- Oliver AJ (1999) *Risk Adjusting Health Care Resource Allocations: theory and practice in the United Kingdom, The Netherlands and Germany.* Office of Health Economics, London.
- Oregon Health Services Commission (1991) *Prioritisation of Health Services.* Oregon Health Commission, Salem.
- Pickin C and St Leger S (1993) *Assessing Health Needs Using the Life Cycle Framework.* Open University Press, Buckingham.
- Popay J and Williams G (eds) (1994) *Researching the People's Health.* Routledge, London.

- Rose N (1989) *Governing the Soul*. Routledge, London.
- Scottish Executive Health Department (2000) *Fair Shares for All. A guide to the final report*. Scottish Executive, Edinburgh.
- Scottish Executive Health Department (2000) *Fair Shares for All. Final report*. Scottish Executive, Edinburgh.
- Symposium (1990) The ethics of resource allocation. Proceedings of a symposium at the University of Manchester during the Annual Scientific Meeting of the Society of Social Medicine, Sept. 1989. *Journal of Epidemiology and Community Health*. **44**: 187–90.
- Tannahill A (1985) What is health promotion? *Health Education Journal*. **44**: 167–8.
- Tones K and Tilford S (1994) *Health Education – effectiveness, efficiency and equity*. Chapman and Hall, London.
- Townsend P and Davidson N (1982) *Inequalities in Health: The Black Report*. Penguin, London.
- Whitehead M (1992) *The Health Divide*. Penguin, London.
- Wilkinson J (ed.) (1988) *Christian Ethics in Health Care*. The Handsel Press Ltd, Edinburgh.
- World Bank (1993) *World Development Report 1993: investing in health*. Oxford University Press, New York.
- World Health Organization (1978) *Report on the International Conference on Primary Health Care. Alma Ata, 6–12 September*. WHO, Geneva.
- World Health Organization (1985) *Targets for Health for All*. WHO Regional Office for Europe, Copenhagen.
- World Health Organization (1986) *Ottowa Charter for Health Promotion. An international conference on health promotion, November 17–21*. WHO Regional Office for Europe, Copenhagen.
- Various (1993) *Rationing in Action*. BMJ Publishing Group, London.

# CHAPTER 6

# Building a vision and changing the world: developing and implementing policy and strategy

*Tony Baxter*

## Introduction

A competent public health specialist needs to be able to understand the impact on health of public policy and to influence the process of the development of policy and strategy. Developing and implementing policy and strategy are key work areas of the public health practitioner.

The purpose of this chapter is to explore some of the competencies required for policy and strategy development and implementation. Some, but not all, of the questions are answered in this chapter and within other chapters of the book.

The chapter concludes with a summary of learning points and further reading.

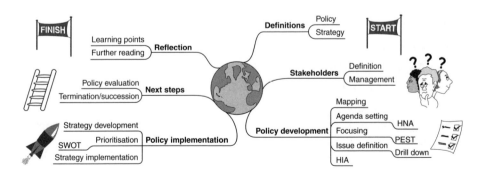

**Figure 6.1:** Mindmap of Chapter 6.[1]

# Definitions

'The creatures outside looked from pig to man, and from man to pig, and from pig to man again; but already it was impossible to say which was which.'[2]

In practice, the terms policy and strategy are often blurred and sometimes used interchangeably. To assist the reader, this chapter has adopted the following definitions.

- A public policy is a course of action or principle adopted or proposed by a government, party, business or individual. It must have been generated or at least processed within the framework of governmental procedures, influences and organisations. A policy describes a broad course of action or principled framework that guides development of strategies. Policies are implemented by a programme of strategies.[3]
- A strategy is a category or type of action to achieve specific objectives. Strategy development cannot take place in a policy vacuum. Strategy is concerned with how aims will be achieved, not with what those aims are or ought to be, or how they are established. Strategy is a term that comes from the Greek word *strategia*, which means 'generalship'. Strategy in the military context refers to the deployment of troops. If the term 'troops' is substituted by 'resources' then the use of the concept from its military sense to other settings becomes clear.

Through the exploration of a case study on disability, which covers a wide variety of agencies and organisations, the reader will explore some of the key competencies inherent in effective influence and development of policy and strategy. I have also used this example because of the importance of disability in society.

The development of policy and subsequent strategies has been defined by several authors as a dynamic process, but one having a series of stages. Although in practice the stages are not often sequential, in this case study they are presented in series to illustrate more readily some of the key considerations.

---

**Case study**

**Developing and implementing policy and strategy for disability as a key component of public health practice**

Dr A works in Bodborough Primary Care Trust (PCT). The trust is in an area of profound socio-economic deprivation. The local borough council's and Bodborough PCT's boundaries are coterminous.

Dr A has been asked to lead the development of local policy for disabled people. He is to chair a local policy advisory group (PAG) comprising representatives from the local NHS sector, local authority and voluntary agencies. The PAG has been in existence for a number of years.

---

# Managing stakeholders

During the process of policy and strategy development, it is good practice to take an active approach to stakeholder management. A stakeholder is anyone who has an interest either directly or indirectly in your work (*see* Chapter 10).

In this particular task, Dr A has two key stakeholders.

- The sponsor – the person or group who allocated responsibility for the work.
- The customer – the end user of the outcomes of the work. Dr A and the group will have multiple customers: for example, local people who will use the services; local voluntary groups; local professionals who will be delivering services.

It is useful to agree performance management arrangements with your sponsor. This may take the form of regular face-to-face meetings or regular reports to committees.

One way to reduce the problems of meeting the needs of multiple customers is to meet regularly with customer representatives who have necessary authority to take decisions on behalf of the group they represent. To some extent, the membership of the PAG fulfils this requirement. The customer representatives are responsible for liaison with those whom they represent.

# Policy development

## Step 1: mapping the territory

---

**Case study – continued**

Dr A reviews the terms of reference and membership of the group and minutes of previous meetings. He discovers that the group developed a policy several years previously. The previous policy aimed high and was based on sound principles but the resulting strategy only delivered some incremental service developments. He speaks to some of the members of the group. From all accounts, the group is dysfunctional with some dominant and disruptive members. Dr A isn't looking forward to his first meeting.

---

**Exercise 6.1**

- How would you prepare for your first meeting as the chair of this group?
- What skills are important in a chairperson?
- How might you influence the behaviour of group members so that all have an opportunity to make effective contributions in this forum?
- What kind of membership should such a group have?

**Case study – continued**

Dr A prepared well for his first session in the chair of the policy group and the meeting went well. The group agreed that a fresh approach was necessary to develop new policy. They agreed that a social model of disability should underpin this. The group decided that the membership needed to be extended to include disabled people and carers.

# Step 2: setting the agenda

**Case study – continued**

The group agreed the aims of the local policy were to enable more independent living for the disabled people in Bodborough, and encourage equality of opportunity by tackling environmental and social barriers in the borough.

**Exercise 6.2**

- How would you develop an agenda that comprises the issues important to such a policy development?
- What sources of information would you explore?

**Case study – continued**

Dr A recommends the group searches for issues relevant to the development of such a policy. He realises that in order to make a robust assessment there are many factors that need to be taken into consideration. Such factors may be identified from information (*see* Chapter 1) available through:

- routinely collected data
- demographic data
- social indicators and social data
- literature reviews
- reviews of existing policies and strategies
- discussions with stakeholders.

He reviews information available on national policy for disabled people and examples of locally produced policies and strategies in other parts of the country. He looks at what epidemiological information is available on disability in Bodborough. He searches for evidence of effective interventions that support the policy aims.

The group chooses to identify issues by using a comprehensive needs assessment approach to take account of these factors. Comprehensive needs assessment looks at corporate views of organisations and individuals, epidemiological information and comparative information (*see* Chapters 1 and 5). Dr A also undertakes a literature review to identify models of service development that have worked in a UK setting, and also to understand the national policy framework relating to disability issues. The results of this work are triangulated (*see* Chapter 9) to identify priority areas.

The following broad themes are identified as being of local concern.

- There are insufficient activities promoting health and well-being in people with existing disabilities, and there is a need to increase activities that prevent disability.
- Access to services is often difficult because of a lack of information and advice on all aspects of disability living. The process of obtaining services through assessment by the appropriate agencies is not well co-ordinated.
- There is no range of housing options on offer to suit individual lifestyles and life stages of people with disabilities.
- There is limited appropriate, flexible and sufficient assistance with personal care and daily living tasks, domestic/homemaking duties and social/quality of life activities to enable individuals to live as independently as they wish.

- Disabled people feel they have limited opportunities to participate in all aspects of ordinary community life, including employment, education, leisure activities, transport and healthcare.
- There are no schemes in place to support training, counselling and advocacy to enable individuals to aspire to and reach their full potential and to take advantage of the available services.
- There is concern among health and social care professionals about the range and capacity of specialist services available to Bodborough residents to help them minimise or overcome disabilities.

# Step 3: focusing on what is important

**Exercise 6.3**

- When developing policy, having identified issues that might be relevant, what factors would you take into consideration that determine what is most important locally?

**Case study – continued**

Having been through a process to identify the broad issues of concern for disabled people in Bodborough, Dr A recognises that the breadth of the agenda means the group have to prioritise areas on which to focus local policy. There are many considerations for the group. Among the issues they have to consider are:

- local and national politics
- the agendas of local organisations
- whether there is any scope for choice
- whether there is consensus about issues and their solutions
- the values underpinning the decision making
- how many people are affected and how are they affected
- the costs and consequences of deciding on a particular course of action.

Dr A thinks that a PEST analysis may be useful in helping to determine how the policy should take account of these factors.[4]

- **P**olitical factors – both big and small 'p' politics. This includes legislative requirements.
- **E**conomic influences – the financial and other resources available in Bodborough.
- **S**ociological issues – demography, trends in how people live and work.
- **T**echnological innovations – new approaches to new and old problems.

The group undertakes a PEST analysis and agrees that local policy should be focused on four theme areas:

- disability prevention and health promotion for disabled people
- improving access to services
- development of specialist services
- improving participation in all aspects of ordinary community life, including employment, education, leisure activities, transport and healthcare.

## Step 4: defining the issues? Turning policy into strategies

**Case study – continued**

Dr A recalls a quote from a book he once read: 'an excellent solution to an apparent problem will not work in practice if it is the solution to a problem that does not in fact exist.'[5]

**Exercise 6.4**

- What techniques might you use to 'drill down' to specific issues that might be amenable to action?
- How would you enable clinical colleagues to inform policy? (*See* Chapter 10.)

**Case study – continued**

Dr A realises this stage is important but challenging because it is as much influenced by principles as facts. Principles can facilitate policy making by providing a viewpoint within which the 'correct' answer is clear. It is important to understand that in complex, multi-agency environments there may be contradictory or competing principles.

The work that the group had done earlier when they agreed to build the policy on a social model of disability made this job easier because all agencies represented on the group had signed up to the same principles. However, agreement still had to be reached on the definition of specific local problems to be solved in the theme areas.

The group chooses to use a technique called 'drill down'.[6] This technique can help to break a large and complex problem down into its component parts, so that plans can be developed to deal with these parts. It also shows you which points you need to research in more detail.

**About drill down**

- Start by writing the problem down on the left-hand side of a large sheet of paper.

- To the right of this, write down a list of points relating to the problem. These may be factors contributing to the problem, information relating to it or questions raised by it.

- For each of these points, repeat the process. Keep on drilling down into points until you fully understand the factors contributing to the problem. If you cannot break them down using the knowledge you have, then carry out whatever research is necessary to understand the point.

By taking this approach, Dr A and the group identify a number of specific local issues within the broad policy theme areas. They identify the barriers to be overcome if the policy is to help disabled people lead more independent lives.

An example of such a specific issue is the lack of information about local housing stock. If the extent to which existing needs for adapted housing were met was unknown, it would be difficult to know how to develop a range of options to meet needs.

# Step 5: health impact assessment. If these issues are tackled, what would the impact be?

**Case study – continued**

The group feels that it is getting close to identifying some strategies that might be employed to deliver the aim of the disability policy. Dr A feels that the group needs to test out some of the proposed changes. He has read about a process called health impact assessment which has been used to assess the impact on health of different policies and actions and he thinks the technique might be useful.

**Exercise 6.5**

- What do you understand by the term health impact assessment?
- What types of health impact assessment are there?
- What steps are involved in health impact assessment?

## Health impact assessment

Health impact assessment (HIA) is a relatively new concept. HIA provides a rigorous way of understanding the potential health benefits and risks of policy and practice.

HIA stems from the understanding that a wide range of different factors affect population health and it is important therefore to assess the impacts of policies and actions which affect these factors and hence impact on health. HIA focuses on equity, sustainable development, participation, and quantitative and qualitative evidence.

HIA can be carried out:

- prospectively (before implementation to help planning)
- retrospectively (after implementation to evaluate)
- concurrently (during implementation to monitor and take corrective action).

There are benefits associated with each type of HIA, but as a technique, it is focused on achieving better results and tackling health inequalities.

The following lists the steps involved in carrying out a health impact assessment.

1 Screening – quick assessment of projects, programmes or policies for their potential to affect health.
2 Scoping – once decided that HIA will take place there is a need to establish a steering group of partners, set boundaries and agree the process.
3 Appraisal – this process involves analysis, population profiling, identifying and reporting impacts and making recommendations on how the impacts should be managed.
4 Decision making – a steering group makes recommendations to decision makers about changes to the original policy proposals in order to minimise the negative and maximise the positive impacts.
5 Monitoring and evaluation – helps to improve HIA process, modify future proposals and assess actual impacts against the predicted effects.

# Policy implementation

## Step 1: setting strategies and tasks

**Case study – continued**

Dr A and the group decide to apply HIA prospectively to the developing policy. As a result of this process, they identify the policy areas likely to have the greatest positive health impacts and minimise negative health impacts.

**Exercise 6.6**

- Once you have identified policy areas to focus developments on, what would you do next?

**Case study – continued**

Dr A and the group recognise that the policy work they have done so far has helped them identify a number of specific objectives. The group must now develop a number of specific strategies to address the agreed areas, and determine actions to deliver them.

Remember: a strategy is a category or type of action to achieve specific objectives. It describes how resources will be deployed to implement an objective.

The group agree the following strategies will have the greatest impact on delivering the Bodborough disability policy.

- Increasing activities that promote health and well-being in people with existing disabilities, and increasing activities that prevent disability.
- Improving access to services by improving co-ordination between agencies to provide information and advice on all aspects of disability living and the process of obtaining services through assessment.
- Improving opportunities to participate in all aspects of ordinary community life, including employment, education, leisure activities, transport and healthcare.
- Improving the range and capacity of specialist services available to Bodborough residents to help them minimise or overcome disabilities.

Dr A and the group break each of the strategy areas into a series of specific actions. For example, a local voluntary organisation has been running a programme called 'Stepping Out' which enables more severely disabled people to access leisure facilities in the community. The group would like to increase the capacity of this programme. This would help meet two of the stated strategies.

At this stage in the work, as chair of the group, Dr A is asked to present a progress report on the policy to his sponsor – the Joint Agency Committee (JAC). JAC has senior board level representatives from all statutory agencies and major non-statutory agencies in Bodborough.

---

**Exercise 6.7**

- How would you prepare a paper with specific policy recommendations to a major decision-making body?
- How would you prepare and deliver a presentation to support your paper?

## Key considerations in producing written reports

- Know what you want to say before you start writing. Gather the information you will need in order to justify what you say.
- Know your audience – use language and technical terms appropriate for your target audience.
- House style – many organisations and meetings have a house style for written presentations to enable the reader to access the most important information and identify decision points. Use such a house style to your advantage.
- Structure your report. Present the information you have in a logical manner that supports your case. Consider prefacing your report with an executive summary. An example of such a structure follows.
  - Summary.
  - What is the issue? Try and make this synoptic and catchy.
  - How big an issue is it? You might consider using a sprinkling of epidemiology here.
  - What works and for whom?
  - What is happening now?
  - What needs to change?
  - What potential options are there (including 'do nothing')?
  - Conclusions.
  - Recommendations to implement chosen options.

## Key considerations in presenting written reports

- Know your audience – use language and technical terms appropriate for your target audience. Try to understand their likely stance on the issue you are presenting.
- Know the house style – ask if visual aids are used to support presentations.
- Know how long you will have to present your report and how long you will have for discussion.
- Don't read your report verbatim. Your audience will have read it and you are unlikely to have time!
- Do present key points for information, discussion and decision.
- Know what decisions you need from your audience and get confirmation of what decisions have been agreed.

---

**Case study – continued**

Dr A has mixed fortunes at the JAC meeting. The overall policy direction is supported, as are the strategies chosen to deliver the policy. However, it is being predicted that the statutory sector financial settlement for the forthcoming year is unlikely to be favourable. This will mean that there will be very little scope for development of services unless they are resource neutral or funded by service reconfiguration. The group is asked to prioritise between the strategies and actions they have identified and present some options back to JAC.

Dr A takes the message back to the group.

---

## Step 2: prioritisation and options analysis

---

**Exercise 6.8**

- How would you help the group identify priorities?

---

**Case study – continued**

The group understand they have only limited resources at their disposal and there are a number of ways they could cut the cake. They are uncertain as to how to choose between localities, between population groups, between disease and dependency groups, between different service or care activities, between different forms of intervention, between different provider agencies.

Because of the array of potential choices the PAG have to make, Dr A establishes a subgroup to determine a simple framework to help prioritise objectives. He realises that there are many possible dimensions to this. The group agree a series of criteria to help them prioritise. The criteria they choose are a mixture of objective, subjective and political.

- Intrinsic – is this an opportunity ripe for development?
- Demand – are people clamouring for a service?
- Need – prevalence, severity, who affected, political concern?
- Net social or economic benefit?

The technique the group use to identify priorities is called a SWOT analysis. SWOT is an acronym for strengths, weaknesses, opportunities and threats. A SWOT analysis focuses attention on the match between what is being proposed and what the external environment needs and wants. In the case of the disability policy, the strengths and weaknesses are those of the proposals, and the opportunities and threats are external.

After much debate, the group agree their priorities for implementation. They consider available options for implementation, and define them carefully based on a number of financial scenarios. They must now present their preferred option or a small number of feasible ones to JAC.

# Step 3: strategy implementation, monitoring and control

**Case study – continued**

In an ideal world, the group would be able to proceed with full implementation of all aspects of the policy. There would be sufficient time and resources available, the policy would be implemented and the desired outcomes achieved, there would be no misunderstandings and all would be co-ordinated like a well-rehearsed orchestra.

However, life in Bodborough is not like that. Unfortunately, finances for development in Bodborough are very limited and local disability services have to compete with many other priorities for funding. As a result, many of the group's aspirations will be unmet.

**Exercise 6.9**

- When you are implementing strategies, what broad types of options are open to you in a situation where resources are limited?

**Case study – continued**

When they review the actions they identified, the group realise that:

- some of these are *resource neutral* and can be implemented fairly easily;
- some can be implemented readily by *reorganising aspects of existing service delivery*, or *negotiating modified objectives* for some service professionals (though this depends on a robust understanding of existing provision) – the membership of the group gives them the power and influences to achieve this
- others require *additional resources*, and Dr A presents outline business cases for these as options for discussion to JAC.

At the end of the financial planning cycle, a modest investment is agreed in disability services and this resource is targeted at two of the group's highest priorities. These are: an extension of the 'Stepping Out' programme to ensure that more disabled people are able to access a wider range of facilities of their choice; and provision of a budget for specialist communication aids for people with sensory impairments and communication difficulties.

Responsibility for delivery of the above actions is allocated to service managers. Delivery targets are set and a reporting mechanism is established through a performance management subgroup of the board.

The outline business cases for developments not chosen are not discarded because they did not get funded this time. From past experience, Dr A realises that opportunities to fund development from outside mainstream funding occasionally present themselves. Such opportunities often have short timescales for submission of funding proposals, so the rejected business cases are kept on file.

Six months after implementation begins, an opportunity for further funding arrives! The government announces a new initiative aimed at increasing investment in health and social care services in the most deprived areas of the country. These areas are called Deprived Area Action Zones (DAAZ). JAC recognise that Bodborough is an area that would be likely to attract DAAZ funding and work together to develop a local bid.

Dr A and the Disability PAG think that the local disability policy could be almost fully implemented if some of the proposed DAAZ funding could be used to implement the strategies that the group developed. In addition, the evaluation component of DAAZ status would provide a unique opportunity to assess the impact of policy implementation.

Bodborough becomes a first-wave DAAZ site and disability is chosen as one of the local theme areas. The policy development work undertaken by Dr A and the PAG has enabled this additional, and unexpected, resource to be accessed opportunistically for the benefit of Bodborough people.

# Step 4: evaluation

---

**Exercise 6.10**

- How would you evaluate the development and implementation of a policy?

---

**Case study – continued**

Using DAAZ funding, Dr A designed the evaluation of the policy to look at the:

- structure – how the policy was developed and implemented
- process – whether the strategies delivered their objectives
- outcome – whether the policy achieved its desired health impacts.

---

## Avoiding pitfalls in evaluating policy

- Are the objectives clear and specific?
- Are success criteria defined?
- Are processes to measure success criteria established?
- Is there a clear threshold beyond which the policy could be described as successful?
- Are there any unexpected side effects of the policy?
- Can you separate the impact of the policy from other influences?
- How sensitive are your processes for monitoring and evaluation?
- Is the impact of the policy distributed as expected?

HIA has already been described as a technique that may help in this arena.

---

**Case study – continued**

**Key learning points**

Dr A is a reflective practitioner and he looks back on what he has learned about the development of policy and strategy as a result of his work on disability in Bodborough.

- He understands that a policy describes a broad course of action or is a principled framework that guides development of strategies. Policies are implemented through a programme of strategies.
- When developing policy, it is important to understand the territory and prepare well for your participation in policy development fora.
- Dr A was aware throughout the development and implementation of this work of the importance of managing key stakeholders. He had two key stakeholders to engage – his sponsors and his customers.
- Once the overarching principles of the policy have been adopted, it is important to use a robust method to set the agenda or broad courses of action. Dr A used a comprehensive needs assessment to achieve this.
- After clarifying what is relevant within the policy context, the next step is to identify what is most important so that the development can be focused. There are ranges of internal and external factors that need to be considered here. Dr A and the group used a PEST analysis to help with this process.
- Once the important areas for development are identified, the next step is to define some specific problems to be solved in the different areas. Dr A used the 'drill down' technique to select some issues.
- Health impact assessment is a useful technique to gauge the health impacts of pursuing a course of action. As a result of this process, the group identified the policy areas that were likely to have the greatest positive health impacts and minimise negative health impacts.
- Because resources were so limited, the group used a SWOT analysis to help them determine priorities for action. They then considered various options for implementation, including options that were resource neutral or involved reconfiguration of existing resources.
- Once they decided a course of action, strategies and tasks were set to ensure delivery. Responsibility for delivery of the actions was allocated to service managers. Delivery targets were set and a reporting mechanism was established through a performance management subgroup of the board.
- Dr A had the foresight not to discard plans for developments that were not resourced immediately. Unanticipated opportunities for funding occasionally present themselves – forewarned is forearmed!
- Dr A had always considered evaluation in service settings to be a bit of a luxury. As a result of the opportunity that DAAZ funding offered, he realises evaluation should always be a component of any major project but also knows this may prove difficult to implement routinely.

Dr A feels he has learned a lot from his experiences.

**So is this the end?**

Dr A feels this is the end of the active policy development for disabled people in Bodborough – for now. He ponders what might happen to the policy in future.

The group is proud of the work it has done on developing and implementing the policy. However, group members realise the policy is not permanent and in future will have to be terminated and replaced by a completely new policy, or undergo succession. (Policy succession is more evolutionary than termination – it is where the process and the outcomes of the policy process are shaped by existing policies.) This is because the group knows that problems change, solutions change, resources change and demand changes.

They agree to keep the policy under review and try to determine natural points for succession and termination.

'This is not the end. It is not even the beginning of the end. But it is, perhaps, the end of the beginning.'

Winston Churchill (1942)

# References

1 Mindmap software@MindMaps™ © 1999 MindJET LLC.

2 Orwell G (1945) *Animal Farm*. Seckler and Warburg, London.

3 Hogwood B and Gunn L (1984) *Policy Analysis for the Real World*. Oxford University Press, Oxford.

4 Iles V and Sutherland K (2001) *Organisational Change: a review for health care managers, professionals and researchers*. National Coordinating Centre for NHS Service Delivery and Organisation, London.

5 Steiss AW and Daneke GA (1980) *Performance Administration*. Lexington Books, Lexington, MA.

6 http://www.mindtools.com/pages/article/newTMC_02.htm (drill down: accessed 17 January 2002).

# Further reading

The following is a short list of reading resources that you should add to as your reading expands.

- Buzan T (1989) *Use Your Head*. BBC Books, London.
- Fiedler B and Twitchin D (1990) *A Framework for Action: developing services for people with severe physical and sensory disabilities*. Living Options in Practice, London.

- http://www.mapnp.org/library/ (Management Assistance Programme for Nonprofits, accessed 16 January 2002).
- Jessop E (2001) Effecting change in meetings. In: D Pencheon, C Guest, D Melzer and JA Muir Gray (eds) *Oxford Handbook of Public Health Practice*. Oxford University Press, Oxford.
- Jessop E (2001) Writing to effect change. In: D Pencheon, C Guest, D Melzer and JA Muir Gray (eds) *Oxford Handbook of Public Health Practice*. Oxford University Press, Oxford.
- Johnson G and Scholes K (1999) *Exploring Corporate Strategy* (5e). Prentice Hall, London.
- Samson Barry H (2000) *A Short Guide to Health Impact Assessment*. National Health Service Executive, London.
- Scott Samuel A, Ardern K and Birley M (2001) Assessing health impacts on a population. In: *Oxford Handbook of Public Health Practice*. Oxford University Press, Oxford.
- Stevens A and Raftery J (eds) (1997) *Health Care Needs Assessment*. Radcliffe Medical Press, Oxford.
- Young TL (2000) *Successful Project Management*. Kogan-Page, London.

# CHAPTER 7

# Working with and for communities to improve health and well-being

*Angela Scott*

## Introduction

My definition of *working with communities*, developed from a number of sources, is as follows.

> The ability to identify appropriate methods of working with communities to increase their control over factors influencing their health and social well-being and to enable their participation in the decision-making process.

This chapter provides a framework for understanding good practice in working with communities to improve health and social well-being in the following ways.

- Actively involving them as partners in all stages of development of intervention programmes and services, from the needs assessment and planning stages through to review and evaluation, and demonstrating the impact of this process on both the way an organisation makes its decisions and on the final outcomes.
- Empowering communities to improve their own health by supporting their understanding of the wider determinants of health and offering choices enabling them to prioritise their agenda.
- Building community capacity by individual development, capacity building within local groups and developing the local community infrastructure.

The chapter comprises the following sections:

- learning objectives
- educational methods
- case study
- key issues/questions arising from the case study

- key issues for working with and for communities
- methods of participation
- exercises
- suggested further reading.

## Learning objectives

By working through the contents of this chapter the reader should:

- have an understanding of the concept of a community
- have an overview of the various methods and approaches to working with communities
- be able to make an informed choice about what methods are appropriate
- work though some of the challenges facing those who work with and for communities
- understand the scope and timeframe associated with this way of working
- understand the conflicts which may arise and consider ways of resolving them
- appreciate the benefits of working with communities.

## Educational methods

It is recommended that the reader utilise the following educational approaches to acquire the necessary knowledge to understand the working methodologies and develop some of the skills and attitudes needed to work with and for the community:

- reading
- attend community groups
- interview people already involved in this way of working
- visit projects
- set up project plans
- look at other codes of practice/principles of involvement
- write out your own set of principles for community involvement.

## Background to the case study

## Developing a geographically located community project to tackle health inequalities

The need to include community development within the framework of public health competency is based on the recognition that social approaches are an important part of a range of solutions which need to be developed to reduce inequalities in health.

Evidence exists that, along with economic and environmental considerations, social approaches may have considerable scope for improving health
and reducing the major public health problems such as heart disease, cancers,
mental health and accidents. The Acheson report on inequalities in health
summarises the evidence and makes recommendations for future policy and
strategy development.[1]

Social approaches underpin a wide range of government-funded initiatives
designed to address health inequalities, including the National Strategy for Neighbourhood Renewal.

Participation of the community in the planning and implementation of
projects is an important principle. The WHO Declaration of Alma Ata states:
'The people have the right and a duty to participate in the planning and implementation of their health care.'[2]

The case study is a construction using real-life issues distilled from years of
practical experience. It is designed to illustrate the wide range of practical problems encountered in community development work. It is based upon developing
a response to a national initiative which involves setting up a geographically
based project with the potential for tapping into substantive funding. The case
study illustrates the processes involved and the learning is applicable to any funded
initiative such as Sure Start, Neighbourhood Renewal or New Opportunities
funding.

---

**Case study**

**'Imagine Us': the Lendon initiative**

Dr Johnson has been asked to lead on the development of the 'Imagine Us'
project, which is to be based in the Lendon area.

Lendon is a small urban area on the outskirts of a large Northern
town. It has been informed it is eligible for a very substantial grant of
both capital and revenue monies, over a five-year period, to address health
inequalities.

The *criteria* which the project bid should meet in order to secure the
grant are as follows.

- The project should be innovative.
- It should be based on identified need.
- It should be produced in consultation with the community.
- It should be managed by a local board comprising two-thirds com-
  munity member and one-third statutory agencies.
- The initial proposal should be produced within six weeks with a full
  business case four months later.
- Include how the proposal will be evaluated.

- Indicate what additional resources will be put into the project by way of matched funding and/or support in kind, i.e. the local resources that will be used, up to an equivalent value – 'matched' – to those available from the grant.

As the grant is part of a much larger regional programme, the project proposal will take about six months to be approved and additional information will probably be needed during the process. It is expected that the notification of the grant will, therefore, not be for another 15 months but spending will need to start as soon as approval is given.

Lendon has several small shopping areas and hosts a twice-weekly market. There are very few sports and leisure facilities in the vicinity and the primary care premises are small and out of date. There are several disused buildings, including an old church and a community hall. The only new purpose-built building in the area is the primary school, which has a large playing field attached. There is also an adjacent area of wasteland.

There is higher than average unemployment in the area, due to the decline of the heavy industry in the region and lack of investment in new industry in recent years. The population has a higher than average mortality due mainly to coronary heart disease and lung cancer. There is also an increase in morbidity among the older male population mainly due to their past employment.

The percentage of smokers is high in the older male population but also among young women. The local police are concerned about the level of domestic violence and the levels of drug abuse and are keen to work with other agencies to tackle the problems they encounter.

There is limited social housing in the area and the perception among the established families is that their youngsters have difficulty getting council accommodation as they feel it is allocated to problem families from the town.

The school has a good reputation with parents and carers. Although unauthorised absences are higher than the national average, they are generally lower than those in the neighbouring schools and the figures are steadily improving. There has also been a measurable increase in the educational standards and the school has raised its attainment levels in Key Stage 1 and 2 in both Mathematics and English.

The children transfer at 11 to the comprehensive school in the town but very few of the youngsters go on to further education.

The teenage conception rate is high and most conceptions result in pregnancy. The young mums with their babies tend to be supported by their extended families.

Apart from the smoking figures there is no other lifestyle information available and much of the health and social data are incomplete and inaccurate.

There are a few active community groups in the area and a small group of mothers have set up an anti-drug-abuse project with the support of the primary care team. It attracts a small amount of funding from the voluntary sector.

There is also a strong church group, which meets on a regular basis to try to address some of the needs of the local population. This group has achieved some very successful results but is viewed with suspicion by many members of the community.

The local politicians are active in the area and have a lot of local knowledge, as do the professionals working there. All have very clear views as to what is needed in the area, but their opinions are very often at odds with each other.

The community has been consulted several times in the past but because of shortage of resources very little has been done. Many of the more active members of the community are of the opinion that the results of the last consultation had not been reported back appropriately.

## Key issues/questions arising from the case study

This case study presents a range of issues, which need to be considered by Dr Johnson and his team, around involving the community in the development of the project proposals. These include the need to:

- define/identify the community
- be clear about what or who is driving the intervention
- identify what the benefits are to the community
- ensure that the process is as open as possible
- consider how they will manage the conflicts of interest within the community
- consider what needs to be done and at what stage
- consider how they will manage community expectations
- plan for sustainability and consider how this can be achieved
- consider the health gain from the intervention and how this will be measured
- consider the importance of cost effectiveness
- challenge the community and organisations' perceptions
- consider how far the project will be able to meet the needs of the community
- consider how the task will be achieved with limited time and resources.

# Key issues for working with and for communities

## What is a community?

The word community can be used to convey a variety of concepts. It can be applied to either a geographical area or to groups with a common interest.

A geographical community or a community of place describe a location in which the residents appear to have some shared sense of belonging and interdependency. They can be applied to housing estates, a village or a larger rural area.

A community of interest relates to a group of people who have common interests or needs. For example, it can be a group of people with a disability, a group of teenage parents or a group of volunteers.

Communities of interest can be groupings either within or across geographical communities.

The shared sense of belonging and interdependency may not always be positive. The regular diet of community interaction served up by television 'soap operas' may be exaggerated but it serves to illustrate the point.

In approaching an understanding of a community it is helpful to categorise the basis for the shared sense of belonging and interdependency.

---

**Meaning of community**

- Community as *heritage* – expressing a common cultural tradition or identity, a sense of continuity and belonging.
- Community as *social relationships* – interrelationships, reflected in kinship, neighbourliness, mutuality and social interaction, often linked with the residential base.
- Community as the basis for collective *consumption* – linked with the needs or demands of groups or neighbourhoods for local public goods, such as transport or play facilities.
- Community as the basis for the most *effective provision* of local public goods, whether by private or voluntary sectors, including the community itself.
- Community as the source of *influence and power* from which is derived empowerment and representation, whether through formal or informal, representative or participative channels of political action.
- The converse to this is community as a shared sense of *powerlessness and alienation.*

*Source*: H Russell.[3]

---

# What is community participation?

Community participation describes the process of seeking to involve people in the decisions and actions in issues affecting their lives. There are traditionally three main levels at which this participation may take place.

1 Working with individuals and groups within the community.
2 Enabling local people and groups to participate in the development and delivery of services at an operational management level.
3 Engaging with groups' local organisations and community representatives to empower them to participate at a strategic level.

The extent to which this participation is passive or active is best described as the 'ladder of participation' as developed by Sherry Arnstein.[4] The lower rungs represent passive involvement, with the highest rungs describing community-run projects.

| The 'ladder of participation' | |
| --- | --- |
| Community control | |
| Delegated authority | Degrees of citizen power |
| Partnership | |
| Involving | |
| Consulting before decisions are made | Advisory capacity |
| Consultation after decisions are made | Rubber stamping |
| Informing | Tokenism |
| Participation in promotion events | Decoration |
| Adapted from the work of Arnstein.[4] | |

This model may be viewed as a hierarchy, with participation at the highest level being aspired to. However, this may not necessarily be the case and participation should be appropriate to the need of the community, the wider circumstances and the impact on the desired outcomes.

Ask the following three key questions.

- Is it desirable?
- Is it feasible?
- What will the impact be?

# What is community development?

Community development aims to empower the people within the community to increase their control over the factors which affect them. This is referred to as building social capital.

It includes the development of social networks and contact systems and increasing the knowledge and skills of the population. It also covers such concepts as trusting others and feelings of safety and self-esteem.

# Regeneration

Many areas, like the one described in the case study, suffer from increasing deprivation. Lack of employment is the underlying cause of much of this decline but deprivation generates other social problems such as: increase in crime, drugs, poor health and low educational attainment. There is also a problem of poor service provision with poor housing and poor and lack of adequate childcare. The interplay of all these factors results in a rapid downward spiral with increasing inequality between areas.

Regeneration seeks to halt this decline, reverse it and prevent it from recurring.

Reviving the economy and increasing employment have to be at the centre of any regeneration but also as part of a wider overall strategy.

If people in deprived neighbourhoods are to benefit from increasing employment opportunities they need help to compete for available jobs. They need to be reskilled, re-engaged and remotivated through being matched to appropriate jobs and in developing an understanding that work pays.

While neighbourhoods will not improve without jobs, the other social problems also need addressing.

The government's National Strategy for Neighbourhood Renewal, produced by the Social Exclusion Unit, identifies four key areas for development:

- reviving local economies
- reviving communities
- ensuring decent services
- leadership and joint working.

## Partnership working

Tackling the problems of deprived communities requires effective partnership working at all levels (*see* Chapter 4). Clearly the services need to work together and with the community but also need to work with other organisations in both private and voluntary sectors as well as faith groups and ethnic minority groups.

Good communication is an essential part of partnership working and clear lines of communication should be set up which recognise and use existing mechanisms. Training and support may be needed to enable people to participate as equal partners.

## Strategic leadership

It should be noted that all of the key leadership abilities described in Chapter 8 are required to work in this way.

# Methods of participation

A range of methods is available and the following is not an exhaustive list (details of the techniques are not included here):

- individual interviews
- focus groups
- discussion groups
- public fora
- setting up management groups
- setting up task groups
- attendance at meetings of community groups
- presentations
- questionnaires
- activity-based sessions
- use of art
- conferences
- publicity
- competitions
- use of email and Internet
- involvement of key community stakeholders
- marketplace/stallholder events
- feedback from professionals working in the area
- Nominal Group Technique.

# Exercises

Working with and for communities is a complex and dynamic area of work requiring skill, patience and objectivity. Observing and participating in existing and developing projects is the most effective way of developing these skills.

There are many examples of good practice around and good practice guides are available. Some examples relate to specific topic areas such as coronary prevention programmes while others consider the wider equality agenda. Working with children and young people has not been considered specifically in the case study although the work would include them. Currently, there is a lot of information available in relation to working with and involving young people.

The following exercises are suggested as examples for developing the skills needed for working with and for communities.

---

Exercise 7.1

- Choose an example of good practice and arrange a visit. Ask for information beforehand and develop a set of questions before the visit. Use the key issues/questions arising from consideration of the case study as a starting point and ask what the problems are.

- Develop your own set of principles/guidelines for working with and for communities and compare these with others.

- Select a project which has been published and undertake a critical review.

- Prepare a 20-minute presentation on the difficulties and benefits of this way of working.

- Look back at the case study and imagine you have been allocated a small amount of funding to develop a community intervention. Plan how you would involve the community in developing a proposal for using this money.

- Choose an example of good practice in working with young people. Consider the key issues. Would this differ from working with adults? Would your code of practice be different?

---

# References

1 Acheson D (1998) *Independent Inquiry into Inequalities in Health: a report.* Stationery Office, London.

2 World Health Organization (1978) *Declaration of Alma Ata.* WHO, Geneva.

3  Russell H (1997) Poverty and community. In: AR Morton (ed.) *The Future of Welfare.* University of Edinburgh, Edinburgh.

4  Arnstein SR (1971) Eight rungs on the ladder of citizen participation. In: BA Cahnse-Passett (ed.) *Citizen Participation: effecting community change.* Praeger, New York.

# Further reading

The following is a short list of books which may be useful as a starting point for further study. They cover some of the different issues in more detail.

- Cutler D and Frost R. *Taking the Initiative: promoting young people's involvement in public decision making in the UK.* Carnegie Young People Initiative, London.
- Graham H (ed.) *Understanding Health Inequalities.* Open University Press, Buckingham.
- NHS Health Development Agency. *Assessing People's Perceptions of their Neighbourhood and Community Involvement (Part 1): a guide to questions for use in the measurement of social capital based on the General Household Survey module.* NHS Health Development Agency, London.
- Regional Director of Public Health for North West England (2000) *Communities Developing for Health.* Regional Director of Public Health for North West England.
- Russell H with Killoran A. *Public Health and Regeneration: making the links.* Health Education Authority, London.
- Social Exclusion Unit. *National Strategy for Neighbourhood Renewal: a framework for consultation.* Social Exclusion Unit, London.
- Social Exclusion Unit. *Preventing Social Exclusion.* Social Exclusion Unit, London.

# CHAPTER 8

# Strategic leadership for health

*Frada Eskin*

## Introduction

This chapter explores strategic leadership within the public health domain and as identified within the Faculty of Public Health Medicine standards document.[1] Public health professionals are primarily concerned with managing the changes required to improve the health of a defined population. Managing change demands focused leadership ability, i.e. the ability to articulate a vision of the future, to bring together the appropriate team of people to turn the vision into a strategy for action and to motivate that team to accomplish the tasks necessary to achieve the required changes.

Strategic leadership for public health is a competence – the ability to achieve a defined goal. This in turn comprises a specific set of skills and knowledge culled from a variety of fields. Additionally, the ability to provide public health strategic leadership requires specific personal attributes – creativity, the desire to be a leader, a mission to make a positive difference in the world, stamina, perseverance, a sense of humour, tact and charm. Not everyone has the capacity or the will to lead. Neither is it necessary to be a leader in order to achieve positive change. Leaders need followers and it is just as important to be a skilled follower.

The components of strategic leadership competence are exemplified in the case study described below and will be explored and supported by suggested tasks to enable readers to develop an awareness of the nature of effective strategic leadership.

By the end of this chapter, readers should be able to understand the implications of strategic leadership and its dimensions, but they will not necessarily be able to lead in practice. Many people possess the appropriate knowledge and skills but have no motivation to put theory into practice.

Public health professionals need to understand strategic leadership and its primary role in the success of public health practice. They also need to be clear about their own capacities and abilities. This chapter is designed to support these needs.

# Learning objectives

The learning objectives of this chapter are as follows:

- **To understand strategic leadership and different models of leadership as applied to public health practice.**
  There are a variety of theoretical models of leadership (*see* further reading at the end of this chapter) and it is important to be aware of these models. At the same time it is necessary to develop an understanding of the importance of personal leadership style. Although leaders develop preferred styles, different situations require different leadership styles and therefore everyone needs to be able to call on a leadership style appropriate to a particular situation and the individuals involved. It is also important to recognise that specific health systems value particular leadership styles which may differ according to cultural values.

- **To understand the role of vision in the development of a strategic plan.**
  Some individuals have the ability to see how the future could be and how to change the existing situation to achieve the change. Those who have vision are not necessarily leaders. As has already been noted, other attributes are required to support visioning expertise. However, without the ability to vision the future, no change is possible. Therefore, a prime requisite for strategic leadership is the ability to see a future better than the current situation. It is probably not possible to teach anyone to vision the future, but it is possible to enable those who can vision to focus on the key issues.

- **To understand the importance of a multidisciplinary approach to strategy development and problem solving.**
  Although it is possible for lone individuals to make key changes at local, national and international level, the modern idiom is multidisciplinary teamwork. Although time consuming, it is the best means of gaining co-operation and, if done well, can achieve lasting, positive change (*see* Chapter 10, pp 217–21).

- **To understand the importance of and the skills required to develop, motivate and manage a multidisciplinary team in the furtherance of strategic goals and action implementation.**
  Developing and managing a multidisciplinary team requires a wide variety of skills. Teams vary in size and may comprise more than ten people. Consummate leadership expertise is required to manage this size of team. Prerequisites for success include a common goal, a willingness to work together, established ground rules for behaviour and, above all, the right leadership. The most effective examples of good teams are probably to be found in the sporting arena. The least successful are probably to be found in healthcare. The reasons for this are considered later in this chapter (*see* Chapter 10).

- **To understand how groups work and to manage their differences effectively.**
  Groups have a life of their own. A group is more than the sum of its individuals and there is a large body of knowledge regarding the working of groups and teams (*see* further reading at the end of this chapter). As most of the work to achieve strategic change is executed within groups, all public health professionals need to have an in-depth knowledge of groups and how they work.
- **To understand the importance of communicating vision and strategic direction to a wide variety of professions and disciplines and to be able to articulate these both orally and verbally.**
  Having said that not everyone is a visionary, there are many potential visionaries who are unable to persuade others of the value of their visions through their inability to communicate. Leaders who succeed have the ability to communicate across a wide variety of fields and hierarchical levels. The ability to enable others to see what you see is determined by a number of factors. The prime factor is the skill of painting pictures with words so that everyone can see the same scene. Otherwise, you may be seeing a horse, but your next-door neighbour may be seeing a camel!
- **To grasp the importance of understanding the health system within which one functions and how to use it effectively to implement change.**
  Health status and healthcare do not function in isolation. They are the outcome of the way in which a society's government operates and how it views its population. Health is a political issue and as such is dependent on government action, the finances allocated and the personnel available to focus on health. In order to function effectively, public health professionals need to understand how societies work, how government evolves and how health and social systems fit within the wider political framework. Without this understanding, public health professionals are impotent to make change.
- **To understand one's own strengths and weaknesses and the importance of taking the long-term view.**
  Another prerequisite for effective strategic leadership is self-knowledge and the willingness to enhance strengths and to obviate weaknesses. Self-development is an essential component of developing leadership expertise. There are many examples of leaders who quite patently suffer from a lack of self-awareness and the ability to endear people. Most of these are political leaders who work through the power of fear. Others find themselves in leadership positions by default. However, whatever successes are achieved are usually short-lived and are unlikely to accomplish positive change.
- **To understand the importance of reconnaissance and of comprehensively mapping the system, its protagonists and antagonists.**
  Good military leaders sweep the skies and assess the situation before sending in their troops. This is appropriate for all forms of leadership, whether in

commerce or the NHS. It is absolutely vital to find out what are the obstacles and smooth pathways before setting off on a strategic road. And there will still be surprises!

- **To understand the importance of gathering allies and supporters and of appreciating others' viewpoints.**
  Effective leaders know the importance of gaining allies and supporters. There is nothing so lonely as rising to speak at a meeting and finding that there is no help from the audience. One of the most powerful forces for change is to be surrounded by a strong, committed multidisciplinary group who will give you their loyal support.
- **To understand the importance of managing the media.**
  The media are extremely powerful because the majority of the population believe that the things which are published in a newspaper or broadcast on airwaves are true. This means that the media must be treated with respect and nurtured as allies.

  The most important lesson to be learned in all of this is that the media are more powerful than public health professionals and cannot be ignored. The media can be a force for good if nurtured and shown respect. It should also be remembered that the media can destroy months and years of work.

# Key issues in strategic leadership

There are a number of key issues to be considered.

- **The purpose of strategic leadership in public health.**
  It is important to understand the role of strategic leadership within the public health field. The essence of leadership is to enable the achievement of particular goals. In public health it is to achieve the change required to improve the health of the population.
- **Leadership development.**
  It has already been noted that not everyone can be or wishes to be a leader. However, unless public health professionals have the ability to assume a leadership role it is unlikely that public health goals can be achieved. Therefore, all public health professionals need to acquire leadership expertise. To become a leader requires both an understanding of what this means as well as practical experience under guidance.
- **Evaluation of progress.**
  The importance of monitoring and evaluating leadership ability is paramount in the process of developing public health expertise. All successes and failures need to be examined, interpreted and the strengths and blockages identified. This will enable effective learning.

# Case study

## Developing a strategic framework for a comprehensive occupational health service in Bunthorpe

This case study illustrates the importance of strategic leadership in public health and how this can accomplish progress with a very diverse group of people not always pulling in the same direction.

Occupational health is a key public health issue although it is not always incorporated into mainstream public health practice. Most people in any society are engaged in work outside the home during their adult life. If the health status of a population is the outcome of the interaction of its individuals with their total environment then the working environment must play a major part in determining the health of workers and their families.[2,3] There is a very large body of evidence to support this statement.

Although work can be a positive force in people's lives, providing both physical sustenance as well as a sense of self-worth, belonging and status in society, the working environment can cause both physical and psychological damage. Therefore, it must be a concern for public health.

This case study demonstrates how public health strategic leadership made a major difference to occupational health in a large city.

## The development stages

The case study is presented in seven stages as follows:

- generating the opportunity
- identifying the problem
- identifying the way forward
- identifying the vision and creating a strategic plan
- integrating into the public health mainstream
- funding issues
- succession planning.

At the end of each stage, key points are indicated, sample exercises are given to guide the reader and significant issues are identified for discussion.

# Generating the opportunity for change

---

**Case study**

The opportunity for action within the field of occupational health in a large British city occurred when I (Dr S), as a newly appointed consultant in public health medicine to the Bunthorpe Health Authority, happened to meet socially and by chance the city's single-handed occupational health physician (Dr K). I had already been involved in some development work with occupational health in a different part of the country and had a clear understanding of the key issues surrounding the marginalisation of occupational health within the public health framework.

At this first meeting, Dr K took the opportunity to bend my ear regarding the low priority of occupational health within the public health agenda. At that time she made some proposals regarding how the occupational health cause could be progressed in the city.

I was receptive to the proposals for a number of reasons. These included previous knowledge of the topic, a personal passion for running with 'lost causes', the need to establish myself in a new job by taking on an issue in which no one else in public health, at that time, was interested. In addition, I also knew that if it were possible to make an impact in the occupational health arena, this would positively change the health of the local population over time. I knew from previous experience that it would be an uphill battle but it was a challenge which interested me. The fact that I had substantial respect for Dr K was also a motivating force.

---

## Key points

The importance of social contact, the ability to communicate, the development of relationships including mutual respect, topic knowledge combined with previous experience, energy to take on 'a lost cause', recognition of a development opportunity, timing.

## Issues for discussion

SEIZING AN OPPORTUNITY

Opportunities need to be recognised. Because Dr S had previously been involved in occupational health issues in another location, she knew the problems and also knew it was possible to do something useful. The occupational physician knew she was the right person to contact. Dr S had published work in this area and had also given talks, at one of which Dr K was present. The opportunity was there for both people. Dr K seized the opportunity at a social event to make contact and to establish a relationship. Dr S had an opportunity presented to her which she could have ignored. For reasons already stated, she chose to take up the issue.

## THE PEOPLE DIMENSION

Dr S knew of Dr K's excellent reputation within the occupational health field. She, too, had published in the field. Dr S respected Dr K's lone fight to develop occupational health in the city. She also liked her. The social interaction was a key stage of the process. The importance of liking and respecting a colleague cannot be stressed too highly as a motivating force in progressing a piece of work.

## POSSIBILITIES FOR A SUCCESSFUL OUTCOME: THE 'IS IT WORTH IT?' FACTOR

Dr S already knew that it was possible to move forward in developing occupational health. However, she also knew that this was because in her previous post she had had the ear of her boss who had access to money as well as being highly respected by his medical and non-medical colleagues. Her power base there was well established. She was not so sure of her position in her new post or if she would be supported sufficiently to be able to move things forward. It was important for her to consider how this issue would be received within her new public health framework.

A successful outcome is determined by a variety of factors. These include:

- a supportive work environment
- the development of a positive power base, i.e. people in powerful positions who support the endeavour
- the availability of finance to support proposed changes
- being in tune with local and national government initiatives
- the demonstration of previous successful outcomes in the same field.

If at least one or two of these factors are in place, a successful outcome is more likely. However, if it appears that taking up the issue at a particular time may be swimming against the tide, then the best action may be to put it on hold.

**Exercise 8.1**

- Describe how occupational health has developed in your country. Who were its champions and how does it relate to public health practice?
- The narrator obviously has a vision for the development of occupational health. Describe what you mean by a vision for a service. Is it necessary to respect someone in order to work with that person?
- Identify a situation in which you have been presented with a strategic work opportunity which you accepted. Analyse this using the framework illustrated in Figure 8.1 as a guide. If you did not take up the opportunity, identify the reasons for not doing so using the framework in Figure 8.1 as a guide.

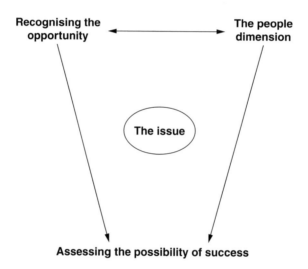

**Figure 8.1:** Assessing the opportunity.

## Identification of the problem

**Case study – continued**

Having spent some time discussing the issues with Dr K, I began to appreciate the complexities involved. There were two key issues at that time (1995). One was the fact that occupational health was not a local priority and the other was the diversity of people and organisations who had or who thought they had a major stake in the occupational health field. This was compounded by the fact that each of these individuals and groups thought they were the leading player. At the time of our first discussions in 1995, no one was really prepared to collaborate. Neither was there anyone prepared to take on a co-ordinating function.

As the city's only occupational medicine consultant, Dr K felt that the weight of responsibility for improving the service was hers. However, she was totally committed to developing a multidisciplinary service and her devotion to the cause was obvious. In addition, she was happy for me to take the lead as she felt that I had sufficient organisational backing to move occupational health onto the mainstream health agenda.

## Key points

Conflict management and conflict management styles, the use and abuse of power, vested interests and hidden agendas, passion, the medical power base.

## Issues for discussion

### PROBLEM CLARIFICATION

When working with a group of people it is absolutely essential to ensure that everyone is explicit about their view of a problem. Previous experience, values, judgements, prejudices, beliefs and culture all have an effect on the way in which individuals view problems and the leader must ensure that sufficient time is spent on teasing out all the elements, views and perceptions in order to reach a common understanding. In addition, vested interests and hidden agendas need to be brought to the surface and dealt with.

### MANAGING CONFLICT

Many people are frightened of raising contentious issues because of the conflict that may arise. However, conflict does not have to be a negative force. Conflict, if managed in a positive way, will be extremely helpful in enabling the development of common understanding in a group composed of a diverse collection of individuals. It can be a motivating force in the process of team development.

PROFESSIONAL ISSUES

Traditionally, the medical profession has regarded itself as being the natural leader in health and healthcare matters. However, there has been a major cultural change. There are now a variety of professions and disciplines working in the field of health and public health who are not prepared to allow doctors to take the lead without specific justification. Medical training by its nature prepares people to take decisions about people's lives, and doctors are used to doing this in the clinical situation – but they are not the fount of all knowledge. Strategic leaders need to take this into account when working towards achieving their goals.

---

**Exercise 8.2**

- Developing a multidisciplinary, multi-agency group is a difficult task. What are the key issues to be taken into account when doing this?

- You have a senior consultant in a group you are developing who makes it clear he does not wish to accept your authority. How would you deal with this to achieve a positive outcome?

- What points do you have to take into account in trying to identify the key issues relating to a problem when working with a new and diverse group of people?

---

# Identification of the way forward

---

**Case study – continued**

We decided that in order to make progress, we needed to gather together all the stakeholders and to identify jointly a way forward. We therefore set up a meeting in September 1995 to include ourselves, the Health and Safety Executive, the Employment Advisory Medical Service, the acute hospital trusts, primary care, health promotion, the occupational health service of the local authority, the university (they run a course for occupational health nurses), occupational health nursing and the Bunthorpe Occupational Health Project (a small organisation concerned with providing a service for workers at primary care level).

The purpose of this meeting was to identify the problem and to find the means of making progress. Prior to the meeting we spent some time discussing who might cause difficulties and how these might be overcome. In addition, I made personal contact with each person either by telephone or by meeting with each of them in order to make sure they understood the nature of the meeting and purpose. The object was to ensure as productive a meeting as possible.

The meeting took place as planned and everyone who was invited participated. The agenda was simple – identification of the key problems, membership of the group and future action.

The outcome was as we (Drs S and K) had hoped. We looked for common ground and found it. Everyone present was anxious to see occupational health as a mainstream service, fully supported by the health community, and everyone wanted to develop a strategy which would enable action to promote occupational health as a key service in the city. My position as chairman of the group was agreed as I was seen as someone who was non-partisan and with a certain amount of power invested in me as a result of my position as a public health physician. It was agreed to meet on a regular basis and to develop an outline strategy. The membership of the group was discussed and it was agreed that we needed to include the local Chamber of Commerce, a trade union representative and a general practitioner.

## Key points

Preparing the ground, finding common ground for dialogue, creating a collaborative climate, the importance of inclusion, management through objectivity, meetings management, the role of chairpersons of groups, appropriate membership.

## Issues for discussion

### OWNERSHIP

If you want to gain commitment to a vision and strategy then those who are involved need to feel that they own the problem. However good you are at problem solving, complex problems have complex answers and in most cases there is no one right answer. Others may have a better solution to offer and the power of the group can be much greater than that of an individual member.

In the modern idiom, all the stakeholders – those people who have a vested interest – need to be involved, respected and their views taken seriously. It is always worth the time and effort required to do this in the context of achieving the vision.

MEMBERSHIP

It is most important to ensure that the membership of a group reflects its needs in terms of both task and process. Membership should include all those people with the knowledge, skills and experience to contribute to the problem solving. In addition, the membership needs to have process skills – managing meetings, chairmanship, team building etc.

It is better to include people than to exclude them. If they find they cannot contribute to the group, they will leave. As a general rule, always invite a willing volunteer, and make sure that you as leader and the rest of the membership know what each other has to offer – and utilise this expertise!

---

**Exercise 8.3**

- Describe a service which you believe needs to be developed. Identify the stakeholders whom you would invite to a joint problem-solving session. Who, of the people involved, are the most likely to resist this process and how might you bring them on board?

- Identify the basis of a successful meeting. What do you need to do to achieve a positive outcome? Describe a success which you have achieved in developing a public health service.

---

# Identification of the vision and creation of a strategic plan

---

**Case study – continued**

In order to ensure the group's progress, and in my new-found position as leading the group strategically, the first thing I had to do was formulate a vision and articulate it to the group so that, despite any differences, we were all subscribing to a common goal. I saw it as my job to do this but to do it in a way in which the rest of the group felt ownership of the vision.

I spent a substantial amount of time thinking through occupational health and the best way of developing a strategic framework which would excite everyone.

In the end, I developed an outline model which I presented to the group at the second meeting (we agreed to meet on a monthly basis). Essentially the elements of this strategic framework comprised the following components (*see* Figure 8.2).

- **Awareness and profile raising** – through the development of a city-wide, multiprofessional, occupational health network, a regular newsletter informing employers and health professionals about what was going on in Bunthorpe, and an annual occupational health conference.

- **Education of health professionals** – especially doctors and nurses – about occupational health and its important role in improving the public health. More input at both undergraduate and postgraduate levels.

- **Central resource centre** – to be based geographically for easy access and to provide a focus for information, support, education and communication for the public, employers and health professionals.

- **Creation of a comprehensive service** – for staff and workers in primary care.

- **Development of existing staff services** – at secondary and tertiary care level.

- **Support for research and development.**

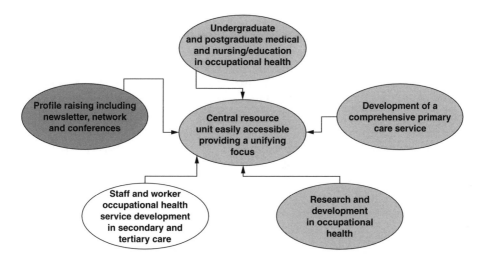

**Figure 8.2:** Strategic framework for occupational health in Bunthorpe.

### Case study – continued

This model was presented to the group at its next meeting and, following discussion, we agreed this would be our focus for the future. We put timescales to each of the elements as well as the amount of funding required. It was agreed that the strategy would be written based on the model and I agreed to produce a first draft.

It took a year to achieve a product which satisfied everyone on the group. As part of our profile development activities, we organised our first conference and launched our strategy at this meeting. We were praised for our attempts but the lack of disagreement worried us. We felt that occupational health was as yet so marginal to other activities, planning processes and service developments that we were being ignored. However, we did not lose heart.

At this point, fortuitously for us, the Health and Safety Executive (HSE) nationally offered some money for local initiatives and our HSE representative proposed to apply for money for a project manager to implement our strategy. He was successful and sufficient monies were allocated both to appoint this project manager on a two-year basis and to develop certain aspects of the strategy, including a regular news bulletin, a series of local occupational health network meetings and an annual conference.

In addition, we applied for and received a small research grant from HSE to survey local businesses for their views about occupational health. The results proved interesting if somewhat predictable. Basically, large firms had services, and small firms, in most cases, said they were not affordable.

It was now that cracks began to show in the group's cohesiveness. The HSE representative, having been able to acquire a considerable sum of money to further the occupational health cause through a national initiative, began to subtly challenge my leadership. It was noted by other members of the group who were equally wary. There were some awkward moments, especially when the project manager was appointed by HSE without me on the interviewing committee. However, the appointment was a success, a lot of activity was implemented and I decided that, as we were going in the right direction, it would be entirely wrong to continue the conflict. Order and harmony were restored.

## Key points

Leadership challenges, the role of finance, conflict of interests, patience, horizon scanning, dedicated personnel, project management, group dysfunction.

## Issues for discussion

### VISION DEVELOPMENT

The purpose of developing a common vision is to create a picture of the future on which to build a strategy – a broad plan of action. Members of a group have their own agendas. They do not always reveal these and, while appearing to be working with you, may well be ploughing their own furrows. It is important to make room for individual need as long as this does not clash with the broad direction of travel. However, the leader needs to pay attention to the group climate and to anticipate impending dissent.

## PATIENCE AS A VIRTUE

Developing vision into an acceptable strategic framework and direction cannot be achieved quickly. If the work is rushed through, it usually fails. The hidden agendas and individual dissent need to be managed so that everyone in the group feels loyal and is prepared to publicly support the outcome. This may take many months and a great deal of hard work. The ground needs to be well prepared and the group needs to develop as a cohesive force despite differing perspectives and personal objectives.

## GROUP COHESION AND TEAM BUILDING

Gathering together a group of people to work on a particular issue is only the first stage of the process. A group can only work well together if there is openness, honesty and trust among all its members. This requires the leader to pay attention and give time to team building – the process of enabling members to become acquainted with each other and to make joint decisions about working relationships, systems and structures.

## LEADERSHIP CHALLENGE

It is often the case that when a group acquires financial resources, there is a surge of interest followed by challenge to the current leadership. 'Horizon scanning', i.e. anticipating trouble, is a very important skill to be brought into play at this time, before the group is irreparably harmed.

## THE GREATER GOOD AND PERSONAL PRIDE

It is a sign of maturity to be able to subjugate one's own needs for the greater good. Effective leadership demands this level of maturity. It is not always easy to give up a particular passion but it may be necessary to do so in order to achieve the broad objectives and to restore harmony.

---

**Exercise 8.4**

- Strategy is the broad plan which puts flesh on the vision. Is it the role of the leader to provide a strategic framework for the group to develop? Would it be more effective to design the framework as a group? From your experience, comment on these questions.

# Integration into the public health mainstream

---

**Case study – continued**

The integration of occupational health within the public health framework was extremely difficult to achieve mainly due to lack of finance and vested interest in other health directions.

Fortunately, the government stepped in with new health promotion initiatives, one focus of which was on occupational health. In addition, health communities were charged with producing health plans known as health improvement programmes and the Director of Public Health was persuaded that occupational health should feature in this document. I was asked to draft a paper for this document and I put in a summary of our strategic plan. At least occupational health was now being viewed as an essential component of the health of the city. Nothing came of this initiative in the short term except that some money was allocated to maintain the Primary Care Occupation Health Project – an organisation represented on the Occupational Health Development Group and dealing with primary care patients and their work problems.

Thus we did manage to push occupational health into the public health mainstream but it did little to help achieve the vision for an integrated, comprehensive service for the city. The group required a lot of input from me, its leader, to keep it enthusiastic and motivated.

---

## Key points

Taking advantage of fortuitous happenings, e.g. changes in government policy.

## Issues for discussion

POLITICAL ASTUTENESS

Sometimes, certain public health issues, even though they are important, do not achieve a high profile. They are not 'glamorous' or 'flavour of the month'. It may be that a particular issue has never had a champion, either in research or in practical action. There may be major financial implications which a government may wish to avoid, or it may be that more pressing and politically attractive issues take precedence.

Sometimes, it is expedient to bide one's time while preparing the ground. Time spent in preparation is never wasted. A key role of a strategic leader is to identify blocks to progress, seek out allies and accrue resources. As has already been noted, achievement of public health goals takes time and patience.

Exercise 8.5

- Identify the factors which are required to support a strategic initiative. How can national government affect the progress of a public health project? What can a leader do to motivate people to continue their work when it appears that there is little support for their activity, even though it is an important public health issue?

# Funding issues

**Case study – continued**

We were reasonably successful in obtaining certain monies to fund the strategic direction. However, the nub of the plan was to develop a central occupational health resource, with a dedicated building, IT facilities, meeting rooms and refreshment facilities. It would serve the whole city and be available to both staff and workers. We needed to raise £250 000 to fund this scheme – and this money was certainly not forthcoming. With the external changes in the National Health Service and the government's move to regionalise, I felt that it might be possible to move away from a city central resource and go for a regional facility. The rest of the group were a little uneasy as they felt that they might lose control over the strategy. At that point I felt that ownership of the strategy had become more important to some people than its achievement, which is what often happens when a group spends a long time developing an idea into practice. I recognised that sowing the seeds of a regional central resource was going to take time and patience and so I kept it as a very low-key issue.

There were alternatives. Industry was beginning to show a major interest in our group and we had senior industrialists asking to join the group. I had every hope that we may have been able to persuade industry of the benefits accruing to them of such a resource.

However, at this point I moved on and left – but before doing so I had spent some time planning for my successor.

## Key points

Changing direction when politically expedient, re-evaluating membership, attracting the right allies, the value of money.

## Issues for discussion

FUNDING AS A SOURCE OF POWER

Power is the ability to make things happen. Availability of funding provides a very important source of power. It enables action. Without funding, it is very difficult to progress any public health initiative. There is little point in spending time developing a strategic framework and direction without paying serious attention to funding issues.

GIVING UP

There comes a time in the life of any initiative when the question of 'How long do we hit our heads against a brick wall?' has to be asked. Enormous effort and energy is constantly expended by substantial numbers of committed and enthusiastic people in developing public health strategic frameworks – the progress of which is consistently blocked by lack of financial resources. The wisdom of this also needs to be questioned in terms of waste of knowledge, skills, energy and time.

---

**Exercise 8.6**

- Identify sources of financial support which may be available for public health initiatives. Discuss the relationship of power and funding in relation to strategic initiatives.

- Strategic development can become an aim in itself. Discuss ways of avoiding this situation.

---

# Succession planning

---

**Case study – continued**

When I knew I was to leave, I wanted to make sure that the group had the right leader and I chose to ask one of the members of the group with vision and political and people skills if he would do this. I felt that these were the skills most needed at this time. We had done all the work on the strategy and now we needed to implement it. He accepted this with alacrity and I left knowing that the group would be well looked after and that occupational health had a champion to ensure progress.

---

## *Key points*

Moving on at the right time, developing the next leader.

## *Issues for discussion*

### INDISPENSABILITY

No individual is indispensable. However, every person is unique and irreplaceable. Leadership should be person independent but it is not. Therefore, in planning for a successor, it is essential to analyse the specific qualities required by the particular group for whom a new leader is being sought. A mature and cohesive group requires different leadership qualities than a new or dysfunctional group. In seeking the right person to lead a group, this analysis will assist a smooth transition.

### CONTINUITY

Groups need continuity. This provides the least disruption and allows the group to concentrate on the task in hand. Continuity can be achieved by selecting a successor at an early stage and allowing that person to gradually assume leadership responsibility while the current leader is still around. Depending on the group and its membership, an internal successor may be the best solution. This is not always the case.

---

**Exercise 8.7**

- 'Effective strategic leadership is person specific.' Discuss this statement in relation to your own experience.
- Describe your ideal public health strategic leader.

---

# In conclusion

The strategic way in which we tackled the occupational health problem in Bunthorpe did make a major difference. Occupational health is now on the mainstream agenda of the health community and work continues towards implementing all the components of the strategic framework.

There are many lessons to be learned from this case. The tasks proposed and the issues explored should enable the reader to achieve the learning objectives outlined above.

# References

1 Documents produced by the Faculty of Public Health Medicine. Refer to website http://www.fphm.org.uk.

2 Sepulveda C (1979) Systemic health planning. *Long Range Planning*. **12**: 62–72.

3 *See* Introduction, Figure A.

# Further reading

The following books are recommended to readers who wish to pursue this topic in more detail. This is not an exhaustive list. There are other very good texts which are too numerous to mention here. Readers are encouraged to seek for themselves.

## Leadership

- Adair J (1998) *Leadership Skills*. Chartered Institute of Personnel and Development, London.
- Adair J (2002) *Effective Strategic Leadership*. Macmillan, Basingstoke.
- Adams JD (1998) *Transforming Leadership* (2e). Miles River Press, VA.
- Bennis WG *et al.* (2001) *The Future of Leadership*. Jossey Bass Wiley, San Francisco, CA.
- Blair J and Fottler M (1998) *Strategic Leadership for Medical Groups*. Jossey Bass Wiley, San Francisco, CA.
- Blanchard K (2000) *Leadership and the One Minute Manager*. HarperCollins Business, New York.
- Conger JA (1989) *The Charismatic Leader*. Jossey Bass Wiley, San Francisco, CA.
- Corbin C (2000) *Great Leaders See the Future First: taking your organisation to the top in five revolutionary steps*. Dearborn Financial Publishing.
- Goleman D, McKee A and Boyatzis R (2002) *Primal Leadership: realizing the power of emotional intelligence*. Harvard Business School Press, Cambridge, MA.
- Handscombe R and Norman P (1993) *Strategic Leadership*. McGraw-Hill Education, Columbus, OH.
- Harvard Business Review (1998) *Harvard Business Review on Leadership*. Harvard Business School Press, Cambridge, MA.
- Heider J (1985) *The Tao of Leadership*. Humanics New Age.
- Jones JH (1994) *Making It Happen: reflections on leadership*. HarperCollins, New York.
- Landsberg M (2001) *The Tools of Leadership*. HarperCollins Business, New York.
- McKenna PJ and Maister DH (2002) *First Among Equals: how to manage a group of professionals*. Free Press.

- Northouse PG (2000) *Leadership Theory and Practice*. Sage Publications Ltd, London.
- Roberts W (1989) *Leadership Secrets of Attila the Hun*. Bantam Press, London.
- Schein EH (1997) *Organisation Culture and Leadership*. Jossey Bass Wiley, San Francisco, CA.
- Sergiovanni T (2001) *Leadership*. Routledge Falmer, London.
- Sims HP and Lorenzi P (1992) *The New Leadership Paradigm*. Sage Publications, London.

## Strategy

- Bandrowski JF (1990) *Corporate Imagination Plus: five steps to translating innovative strategies into action*. Free Press.
- Bowman C (1990) *The Essence of Strategic Management*. Prentice Hall International (UK) Ltd, London.
- Grant RM (2002) *Contemporary Strategy Analysis: concepts, techniques, applications*. Blackwell Publications, Oxford.
- Kotter J (1996) *Leading Change*. Harvard Business School Press, Cambridge, MA.
- Lynch D and Kordis PL (1990) *Strategy of the Dolphin*. Arrow Books.
- Minzberg H *et al.* (2001) *Strategy Safari: the complete guide through the wilds of strategic management*. Prentice Hall, London.
- Morgan G (1997) *Imaginization*. Sage Publications Inc., London.
- Pettigrew A, Ferlie E and Mckee L (1992) *Shaping Strategic Change*. Sage Publications, London.

## Teamwork (*see* Chapter 10)

- Adair J (1986) *Effective Teamwork*. Pan Books, London.
- Gorman P (1998) *Managing Multidisciplinary Teams in the NHS*. Open University Press, Buckingham.
- Holpp L (1998) *Managing Teams*. McGraw-Hill Education, Columbus, OH.
- Katzenback JR and Smith DK (1998) *Wisdom of Teams*. McGraw-Hill Education, Columbus, OH.
- Yeung R (2000) *Leading Teams*. Essentials.

# CHAPTER 9

# Research methods and their application in public health practice

## *Elizabeth Goyder and Darren Shickle*

## Introduction

Many public health practitioners will be involved in research at some time in their work and all public health practitioners need to be able to understand, interpret and apply research findings.

This chapter provides a framework for understanding research methods and how research can be used in public health practice. A study of the use of health services by people with diabetes is used as a case study to illustrate some of the issues arising when undertaking research or using research evidence. Having worked through the material in this chapter, you will be ready to think about applying your learning to developing, and then addressing, research questions in your own practice.

This chapter comprises the following elements:

- learning objectives
- case study
- sections outlining key issues
- exercises
- suggested further reading.

## Learning objectives

After working through this chapter, the reader should be able to:

1 turn a complex public health problem into an answerable research question
2 understand the appropriate use of both qualitative and quantitative research methods

3  conduct a literature review to look for primary and secondary research
4  identify clear aims and objectives for a research project
5  design an appropriate research study to address a specific research question
6  identify the ethical and legal issues which apply to public health research
7  undertake appropriate data collection and analysis to address a specific research question
8  draw appropriate conclusions from research findings and use them to improve health.

# What is 'public health research'?

Because much core public health activity is similar to research activity in that it involves collecting and analysing information, there is scope for uncertainty as to whether some of these public health activities are 'research' or not.

For example:

- Health needs assessment involves collecting and interpreting information about health needs. This is also an aspect of epidemiological research.
- Evaluation of health services and other interventions to improve health is a core public health activity, and is also a major aspect of health services research.

Broadly speaking, if the aim is to produce new knowledge that other practitioners can use in other contexts, you are doing 'research'. If the aim is to use local information directly to improve health locally and the results will not be disseminated further afield, this is probably either 'needs assessment' or 'evaluation'. There is a grey area of work with dual aims. For example, doing a local survey with the main aim of influencing local services may be health needs assessment, but if you publish results from this process that might be generalised to other populations, this becomes research. 'Action research' may also lie in this grey area depending on whether the main aim is to facilitate local change or answer specific research questions.

## Learning objective 1: turning a complex public health problem into an answerable research question

Sometimes a problem or question arises which cannot be answered using readily available local information (*see* Chapter 1). From an analysis of the issues involved, it may be possible to identify a specific research question. For example:

- What are the causes of an increasing prevalence of disease X?
- What are the health effects of environmental hazard Y?
- Is new treatment A more effective than treatment B for condition C?

- What are the reasons for population D having a lower uptake of health intervention E than population F?

Public health is, by definition, a multidisciplinary field and it is not surprising that public health research draws on a very wide range of academic disciplines and their research methods to answer questions. These include the fields of epidemiology, demography, statistics, health economics, psychology and sociology, to name but a few of the more obvious and well-established examples. Traditionally, public health researchers have used epidemiological and statistical methods to find quantifiable answers to research questions. However, qualitative methods, developed principally by social scientists, are now being used to explore and develop the underlying concepts.

# Learning objective 2: understanding the appropriate use of both qualitative and quantitative research methods

Increasingly, the benefits of combining qualitative and quantitative methodologies are being recognised, strengthening research design and the validity of results.[1] The use of information from different sources, often derived using different research methodologies, to address the same research question is generally referred to as 'triangulation'. This allows the researcher to confirm findings and to obtain breadth and depth of information. However, there are also advantages in using one methodology before proceeding to another. In some circumstances, qualitative and quantitative research are part of an iterative process. Qualitative research may be used to generate hypotheses that can be tested on larger samples using quantitative techniques. Qualitative research is also used to explore attitudes in more detail and test reactions to possible interventions. These in turn can be evaluated further using quantitative methods.

Qualitative interviews can help the researcher learn the vocabulary and discover the thinking pattern of the subjects under study. Interviews may provide clues to special problems that might develop in the quantitative phase. For example, the questionnaire might have an illogical sequence of questions that confuses respondents, omit important response options or simply fail to ask critical questions. These insights can be used to develop more efficient quantitative studies, from which the researcher is able to make inferences about the larger population.

Questionnaires typically yield a large amount of data. Qualitative interviews can provide insights about the meaning and interpretation of the results. Follow-up qualitative research can suggest action strategies for problems addressed in the questionnaire.

## Quantitative methods

*Questionnaire surveys* are based on a sample of the population to which they relate.

- *Study validity* is the degree to which the inferences drawn, especially generalisations extending beyond the study sample, are warranted when account is taken of study methods, the representativeness of the study sample, and the nature of the population from which it is drawn.
- *External validity* or generalisability will depend on choosing subjects from an appropriate sampling frame as well as achieving a high response rate.

*Self-completion questionnaires* allow for large amounts of data to be collected from many individuals simultaneously. Statistical analysis allows comparison between groups and subgroups. The ability to detect true differences between groups is dependent on the sample having sufficient power by recruiting adequate numbers of subjects.

Self-completion postal questionnaires are particularly susceptible to low response rates and hence *non-responder bias.* For example, those individuals who return questionnaires are likely to:

- have more time to complete a questionnaire than those who do not
- feel under particular obligations
- have additional motivation because they see the subject as being relevant to them
- have strong views which they wish to express.

There is no agreed figure that is accepted as indicating a *satisfactory response rate.* Unless the response rate is very high (over 90%) you should consider the potential for response bias and try to assess its magnitude. This can be done by examining differences (e.g. in age and sex) between responders and non-responders or, if you do not have any information at all about non-responders, between early and late responders.

*Postal questionnaires* need to be short – otherwise potential respondents become reluctant to devote the time necessary for completion and hence either answer the questions with limited thought or do not return it at all. However, short questionnaires limit scope for testing reliability – for example, by including additional questions on the same subject to test for consistency. Questionnaire length also limits the ability to ask related questions to address various aspects of an issue.

*Quantitative studies* are particularly suited to closed questions. However, quantitative studies are a relatively crude instrument for ascertaining professional views. *Open questions* can be used, allowing individuals to write comments, although this complicates coding. Quantitative techniques also tend to identify concerns that have already achieved some visibility within the community, as opposed to the less visible concerns that lie below the surface.

## Qualitative methods

Qualitative techniques can provide a more in-depth understanding of opinions. *Focus groups* are designed to obtain perceptions on a defined area of interest.

CHARACTERISTICS OF FOCUS GROUPS

- Usually composed of six to ten participants – the group should be small enough for participants to have an opportunity to share their comments, yet large enough to provide a diversity of opinion.
- Composed of people who are similar to each other – homogeneity may be narrowly or widely defined and will depend upon the study and the basis for recruitment.
- Participants usually do not know each other, although in some communities or professional groups it may be difficult to recruit complete strangers – there is a danger that if group members are close friends, or regularly interact, their discussions will be influenced, overtly or covertly, by past experiences or events.

BENEFITS OF FOCUS GROUPS

- Inhibitions are often relaxed in group situations, increasing candour of respondents – people are social creatures who interact with others. They are influenced by the comments of others and make decisions after listening to the advice and counsel of people around them. Quantitative data or one-to-one interviews are not able to capture the dynamic nature of this group interaction.
- The format allows the moderator to probe – this flexibility to explore unanticipated issues is not possible within the more structured questioning sequences of questionnaire-based studies.
- They have high face validity.
- The technique is easily understood and the results are presented in lay terminology embellished with quotations from group participants rather than complicated statistical tables.

DISADVANTAGES OF FOCUS GROUPS

- Groups may be difficult to assemble – the format requires that people give up their time to meet at the same time and place. In contrast, an individual interview can be held at a time and location most convenient to the interviewee.

- Groups can vary considerably, with each group having its own unique characteristics. Because of group idiosyncrasies, it is recommended that enough
  people be included to balance differences between sessions.
- The researcher has less control in the group interview than in the one-to-one
  situation.
- The format allows the participants to influence and interact with each other.
  While this is usually a strength, individual group members may disproportion-
  ately influence the course of the discussion. This sharing of group control
  results in some inefficiency such as detours in the discussion and the raising
  of irrelevant issues. The facilitator must therefore keep the discussion focused
  without biasing the content of the discussion. The facilitator will need to use
  *open-ended questioning*, techniques such as pauses and probes and knowing
  when and how to move into a new topic area.
- Group data are more difficult to analyse – care is needed to avoid taking
  comments out of context and out of sequence. Group interaction provides a
  social environment, and comments must be interpreted within that context.
  It is important to collect data on such interactions. A comment may receive
  significant support from other group members, as demonstrated by non-verbal
  cues, but such group consensus may not be apparent within the transcript.

---

**Case study stage 1**

**A research project that developed from local issues**

The case study for this chapter is based on a real research project carried
out in Leicester in the 1990s. First we consider different ways of addressing
the real questions that arose at that time and then describe the research
actually carried out.

Many general practitioners provide regular routine care for their
patients with diabetes. They are seen regularly, checked for developing
complications and their clinical management reviewed. Other people with
diabetes, particularly those treated with insulin, attend hospital clinics for
regular reviews. The provision of organised diabetes care in general practice has increased over the past 20 to 30 years in the UK, and payments
have been introduced for primary care providers who could show they
were providing structured care. This involves fulfilling a number of criteria,
including having a register of all their patients with diabetes and a system
for ensuring they are reviewed regularly.

It was known that, in the 1990s, service provision was patchy. Not all
general practices provided regular reviews themselves and not all qualified
for the specific payments for diabetes care.

---

**Exercise 9.1**

- Identify three possible research questions that might arise in a discussion of this situation.

---

**Case study stage 1 – continued**

Concerns around the provision of diabetes care in general practice raised a number of questions.

- Why did some practices not provide structured care? What were the differences between practices that did and practices that did not provide care?
- What factors determined which patients were seen regularly in general practice or which patients were seen regularly in hospital clinics?
- If patients were seen regularly in general practice or hospital clinics, were they less likely to need hospital admission? Were they less likely to use emergency services?

---

# Learning objective 3: conducting a literature review to look for primary and secondary research

Often the first step is a search of relevant literature to see if the question has been addressed anywhere else. If you have access to them, it may be helpful to ask specialists or experts in relevant fields to suggest where you might find useful information. You may decide there is enough information in the literature from previous research to address your research question by reviewing or re-analysing this information. In considering the available published information it is helpful to have a suitable framework for critical appraisal of relevant literature (*see* learning objective 8 on critical appraisal). If no adequate answer is found in the research literature, despite a clearly answerable research question, it may be that further research is needed. It is often tempting to rush into data collection but worth remembering as a useful rule of thumb: spend a third of your time on refining the research question, a third on collecting data and a third on analysis and interpretation.

Research which is based on collecting, collating or reviewing other people's research rather than collecting any new data is referred to as 'secondary research'. This may include *systematic literature reviews* or *meta-analyses* of previous findings. A number of useful guides to conducting systematic reviews are available (*see* further reading). This can be distinguished from 'primary research' which involves collecting and analysing new data.

---

**Case study stage 2**

**Developing answerable research questions**

A number of questions about the provision of diabetes care in general practice were generated, for which answers could not be found through literature searching. It was not going to be possible to design a study to answer every question. First, the questions that it might be possible to answer through primary research were considered. It was decided to focus on the relationship between access to preventive care (measured by evidence of review in primary care or in hospital diabetes clinics) and use of acute hospital services.

**The main research hypotheses**

The main research hypothesis could be stated as:

- regular routine review is associated with a reduced risk of hospital admission.

A secondary hypothesis was:

- access to routine review is related to patient characteristics, including age, sex, ethnicity and socio-economic circumstances, as well as clinical factors.

---

**Exercise 9.2**

Consider the main research hypotheses stated above.

- How would you design a study to answer these questions? What are the advantages and disadvantages of these approaches?
- Next read the following section on 'epidemiological study design' and consider which of the types of study described would be able to address these research questions.

---

## Epidemiological study design

There are four main categories of epidemiological study:

- cross-sectional study
- case-control study

- cohort study
- randomised controlled trial.

A *cross-sectional study* examines the relationship between an outcome (usually health related, often a specific disease) and other variables of interest (often described as explanatory variables) within a specified population at one particular defined time. The presence or absence of the various variables are determined in each member of the population or in a representative sample drawn from that population. The relationship between a variable and an outcome can be assessed by measuring the prevalence of that outcome in subgroups defined by the presence/absence (or level) of the variables or by measuring the variable in subgroups with or without the outcome of interest.

A *case-control study* starts with the identification of persons with the disease (or other outcome variable of interest) and a suitable comparison group of persons without the outcome of interest. The relationship of an exposure or risk factor to the outcome is examined by comparing the case and control groups with regard to how frequently the exposure is present. Controls should be similar to cases apart from not having the outcome of interest. Crucially they should have had the potential of being exposed. Case-control studies are retrospective (although it may take time to identify an adequate case series to study). An *odds ratio* is calculated to see whether the group with the outcome of interest were more or less likely to have been exposed than those in the control group. If they are less likely (odds ratio less than one) then the exposure is preventative.

---

**Exercise 9.3**

- In order to answer the research question in this case study, how would you define a case and a control and what would be the 'exposure' of interest? What other factors which are associated with health service use might you need to measure?

---

The exposure here is 'regular routine diabetes review'. The outcome variable within the research question is admission to hospital. The cases are therefore people with diabetes admitted to hospital. The control group would be patients with diabetes who have not been admitted to hospital. Other factors associated with both the likelihood of routine review and the likelihood of hospital admission, such as type of diabetes or presence of other medical conditions, are known as *confounders*. It is important also to measure any potential confounding variables, so that it is possible to draw conclusions about whether a relationship between the exposure and outcome still exists when these potential confounding variables (which could otherwise explain any observed association) have been allowed for in the analysis.

The *case definition* can be made more specific so that it refers only to diabetes-related admissions or admissions within a certain timeframe. It may also be interesting to ask whether patients receiving regular review are less likely to develop diabetes-related complications. A case-control study for such a research question would use patients with a diabetes-related complication (for example, retinopathy) as cases, and patients with diabetes but without any retinal complications as controls.

A *cohort study* involves assessing exposures or risk factors for individuals within a population cohort. The cohort is observed for a sufficient number of person-years to generate enough end points to assess the incidence or prevalence of the outcome of interest (often a disease) in those exposed compared with those not exposed. Cohort studies are usually prospective, but can be retrospective if reliable data on exposure was collected in the past. The *relative risk* is calculated from the data to see whether the exposed group are more or less likely to develop the disease than those not exposed. If they are less likely (relative risk less than one) then the exposure is preventive.

In a *randomised controlled trial (RCT)*, subjects who have consented to participate are randomised to receive (study arm) or not receive (control arm) an experimental preventive or therapeutic procedure or intervention. Both the subjects and those assessing whether there has been a positive outcome should ideally be unaware of whether the subject has received the intervention or not (i.e. both would be 'blind', and hence the term double-blind RCT). If an individual is aware they have been randomised to the intervention arm, they may consciously or subconsciously report more favourable outcomes, because that is what they expect should happen. Thus, rather than control subjects receiving no intervention, they are either given a placebo or current standard practice, such as an alternative therapeutic intervention in widespread use.

ARE RCTs ETHICAL?

Ethical concerns are sometimes raised about randomising to receive no intervention or a placebo. However, such concerns are less valid if current standard practice is used for case subjects in the control arm. In these circumstances, the subjects are not disadvantaged since they would not have received an intervention anyway. It would be unethical to withdraw an intervention where there is evidence of effectiveness. Similarly it would be unethical to perform an RCT where there is conclusive evidence that the intervention to be evaluated is significantly more or less effective or harmful than that in the control arm. It is therefore desirable to conduct RCTs as early as possible in the development of a new intervention. The rationale of conducting the RCT should also be explained as part of the informed consent process.

WOULD IT BE APPROPRIATE TO RANDOMISE INDIVIDUAL PATIENTS TO RECEIVE
REGULAR ROUTINE DIABETES REVIEW?

It would be very difficult to randomise individual patients to receive review or
not. The GP would need to treat patients within the same practice differently
according to whether they have been randomised to receive regular review or
not. Patients within the practice may compare the treatment regimes and question why they are being managed differently. There is a danger of 'contamination',
with patients randomised to the control arm being given some degree of review
simply because it is not practical to treat patients within the same practice
differently. In such circumstances *cluster randomisation* can be used, where the
unit of randomisation is the practice rather than the patient. If a practice is
randomised to the study arm then all of its patients should receive regular
review. In the control arm, no patients would receive review.

WOULD IT BE POSSIBLE TO CONDUCT A DOUBLE-BLIND RCT TO ANSWER
THE RESEARCH QUESTION?

A patient may not know whether routine regular review for diabetes was
standard practice or not; however, it would be very difficult to make the patient
'blind' as to whether s/he has been reviewed or not. Similarly the health professional conducting the review would not be 'blind'. It may, however, be possible
to make the observer 'blind' of whether a subject has had a positive or negative
outcome – for example, by the person recording the admissions using the hospital patient administration system, without having access to the primary care
notes to see how often the patient has been seen by the general practitioner.

   In summary, the advantages and disadvantages of these four study types are
shown in Table 9.1.

## Next steps

Before embarking on a research project it is vital to ask yourself the following.

- Do I have a clear and well-defined research question?
- Is the answer to this question important?
- Can I collect and analyse appropriate information that can answer this
  question?

If the answer to all these questions is yes, and you are keen to conduct a study,
then also ask the following question.

- Can I ensure I have sufficient resources to carry this out? This includes
  money and equipment, but will also include other people's time and expertise

**Table 9.1** Advantages and disadvantages of four study types

|  | Advantages | Disadvantages |
| --- | --- | --- |
| Cross-sectional study (observational, descriptive) | • Usually quick and cheap<br>• Fewer ethical problems<br>• Useful for generating research questions | • Highly prone to bias<br>• No time reference<br>• Difficult to resolve research questions |
| Case-control study (observational, analytical, retrospective) | • Optimal for rare diseases<br>• Can study multiple aetiology of disease<br>• Generally cheaper and quicker to perform<br>• Good for diseases with long latent periods | • Can't calculate incidence unless population based<br>• Prone to recall and confounding biases<br>• Not efficient for rare exposures<br>• Have to rely on adequate notes for previous history, exposure and lifestyle<br>• Temporal relationships may not be clear |
| Cohort study (observational, analytical, usually prospective) | • Optimal for rare exposures<br>• Can study multiple effects of exposure<br>• Can calculate incidence<br>• Adequate data on exposure and confounders more easily obtained as planned in advance*<br>• Minimises recall bias*<br>• Can study temporal relationships* | • Not efficient for rare diseases unless attack rate high<br>• Prone to observer bias<br>• More expensive and time consuming*<br>• Need enough end points to assure statistical power*<br>• Subject to loss of power from loss to follow-up. Possible bias if differential loss (should analyse by intention-to-treat)* |
| Randomised controlled study (interventional, analytical, prospective) | • Optimal for evaluation of effectiveness of therapies<br>• By random allocation, confounders and many biases (known and unknown) are minimised<br>• Placebos and blinding reduces observer bias<br>• Can have various study groups to examine dose-response effect | • Ethical considerations<br>• Healthy volunteer bias reduces end points<br>• Feasibility of finding enough suitable willing volunteers<br>• Poor compliance can lead to loss of power (counter by intention-to-treat analysis) |

* Only applies to prospective studies

and your own time. Time spent on research will always have opportunity costs – so no matter how enthusiastic you feel, don't start collecting data until you are confident you have an adequate study protocol and there is a realistic chance of a successfully completed study.

# Learning objective 4: identifying clear aims and objectives for a research project

The development of clear and specific aims and objectives will clarify the scope of your project and help when you come to identify the details of appropriate methodology. The overall aim describes what the project will achieve in total. The objectives are all the specific individual elements of what the study sets out to achieve, which will together fulfil the overall aim.

---

**Case study stage 3**

**The choice of study design**

Thus, the overall aim of the diabetes admissions study was to explore the relationship between routine diabetes care and hospital admission. The specific objectives that needed addressing in order to fulfil the aim included:

- describing the pattern of routine review for people with diabetes
- describing their pattern of hospital admission
- investigating whether routine review predicted a reduced risk of hospital admission.

A very wide range of study designs could, in theory, address the study hypotheses. The main reasons for not choosing to conduct an intervention study (RCT) or a prospective cohort study were as follows:

- knowledge of the study aims would influence patterns of care during the study period
- it would not be ethical to have a study in which a group of individuals were not receiving regular routine preventive care, when professional consensus is that such care is effective in reducing complications
- it would also take much longer to collect data than with a cross-sectional or retrospective cohort study design.

The main disadvantage of a retrospective cohort design is that it is only possible to use routinely collected information, or rely on recall of previous events (that may be subject to recall bias). However, in this case it was decided that as recalled information could be validated using information from records, a retrospective cohort design would be adequate to address the research questions.

---

## Learning objective 5: designing an appropriate research study to address a specific research question (see above)

The success of a research project will depend on the development of a detailed protocol. The issues to consider and include in the protocol include the following.

- *Aims and objectives* – are these clearly defined and achievable?
- *Study population* – how will you identify the study population? Do you need a 'case definition' to determine who should be included in the study? Will you need to consider sampling strategies? A power calculation is needed to ensure the study population will be large enough to allow you to answer your research question with confidence.
- *Data collection* – for quantitative research, both the explanatory variables (the risk factor or intervention you are interested in) and outcome variables (the medical condition or other health outcome you are interested in) need to be clearly defined.
- *Do you need to pilot the data collection methods?* It may be very important to try out or *pilot* the process if you are using a relatively new method, or an established method or data collection tool in a new setting. Many survey instruments have been developed to measure specific health-related outcomes such as quality of life, disability, anxiety and depression, severity of pain. Both general and disease-specific instruments exist (*see* Chapter 1 and further reading). Developing and validating such instruments is a major undertaking. Where possible, use an established instrument to make it more likely that your results will be valid. You will also be able to compare your results with other studies using the same outcome measures.
- *Data analysis* – it is good practice to know how you intend to analyse your data before you collect it. If you do not have the statistical (or qualitative) skills to confidently plan the analysis yourself, consult an expert at this stage (*not* after you have started collecting data).
- *Study management* – the research process will benefit from involvement of a steering group that can provide feedback and advice at all stages. The steering group should ideally include lay representatives as well as experts in the study topic area and methodology. A realistic timetable for the study should be included in the protocol. Include time for writing up the study findings and getting the results published in peer-reviewed journals.
- *Funding* – the costs of the study should be estimated. Costs include the salaries and overheads for anyone employed on the study, equipment costs and office costs. Don't forget recruitment costs if you may need to advertise a research job and then pay expenses for applicants and interviewers. Don't forget travel expenses related to the project or the cost of organising meetings and attending

conferences to disseminate the study results. There are many sources of advice on research funding opportunities. The appropriate source will depend on the size of the project, the proposed methods and the subject area.

# Learning objective 6: identifying the ethical and legal issues which apply to public health research

Whenever you are collecting information on individuals or populations, there may be ethical considerations. Generally, health service research ethics committees should be asked for approval when information is collected on health service premises or on health service patients. Another practical consideration is that many *peer-reviewed journals* will expect appropriate ethical approval to have been granted for any work they are asked to consider publishing.

In the UK, Local Research Ethics Committees (LRECs) or a Multi-centre Research Ethics Committee (MREC) for larger studies must be consulted if the research involves:

- NHS patients (i.e. subjects recruited by virtue of their past or present treatment by the NHS), including those treated under contracts with private sector providers
- foetal material and IVF involving NHS patients
- access to records of past or present NHS patients
- the use of, or potential access to, NHS premises or facilities (including NHS staff).

The two main ethical concerns with research ethics are:

- informed consent
- confidentiality.

## *Informed consent*

The first step in the process of seeking informed consent is determining whether the subject is able to give consent. In order for a patient to be judged competent or to have the capacity to make autonomous decisions regarding participating in the research, a potential subject must be able to comprehend and retain information pertinent to the decision, especially any consequences of being or not being part of the study. Competence can be difficult to determine. Even individuals who are not fully legally competent, e.g. due to age or mental illness, are capable of expressing rational preferences. In law, children aged 16 or 17 are judged competent regarding their healthcare decision making, and in certain circumstances, children even younger can be judged competent. Following the Gillick case, children under 16 may be judged competent.[2] However, it is still necessary to judge carefully whether or not the child fully understands the implications of his/her decision, and the legal guardian should still be involved in the consent process.

*Disclosure* is the process in which the researcher provides the information to the potential subject necessary for that person to decide whether to participate in the research. Disclosure should inform the subject adequately about the study and what it involves, the benefits and risks and how the results will be used. The goal is to disclose information that a reasonable person needs in order to make an informed decision. This sharing of information encourages interaction between the researcher and subject, building up the relationship that will continue throughout the study. Disclosure is an ongoing process and will need to be repeated as appropriate.

In the simplest terms, in order for a patient to be able to give informed consent, the patient must be able to understand to what s/he is consenting. This lays the burden on the researcher to provide adequate yet understandable information. LRECs frequently require that subjects are given sufficient time to absorb and think about the information before deciding whether to give consent. LRECs may require written information to be in the form of 'questions and answers'.

- What is the purpose of the study?
- What will be involved if I agree to take part in the study?
- Can I withdraw from the study at any time?
- When and where will the research take place?
- What other information will be collected in the study?
- Will there be effects on my treatment?
- Will the information obtained in the study be confidential?
- Will anyone else be told about my participation in the study?
- What if I wish to complain about the way in which this study has been conducted?

A potential subject should be free to make a decision as to whether or not to participate in the research without any undue influence. There must be a balance between the giving of advice and allowing the person to make his/her own decision. For a person to be coerced into participating in a study, there must be a credible threat attached. *Coercion* negates an individual's ability to make an autonomous decision. *Persuasion* is less powerful. This is where a subject is convinced to participate, perhaps against his/her first instincts, through the arguments presented to them. *Manipulation*, on the other hand, is neither coercive nor persuasive. Information is presented to the subject in such a way as to direct him/her, through deception, toward a set of actions. While coercion and manipulation should not be used, researchers may persuade people to participate; however, subjects must be left to give or withhold consent as they wish. Patients' willingness to volunteer may be affected by a sense of obligation to 'repay' the health professionals caring for them by assisting in their research. The voluntary aspect of consent is further affected if patients perceive that the quality of care they receive may be affected if they are seen to snub those responsible for their care. There may be similar problems when conducting research in occupational health, if an employee feels coerced by an employer.

Once the preceding elements have been met then informed consent can be given. Consent may be oral or written. LRECs will usually require a written signature (which may need to be witnessed) to demonstrate that consent has been given. This in part also protects the researcher. A signature does not guarantee informed consent, however. If consent is oral, then it will be more important for it to be witnessed. For research purposes, explicit consent is usually required. However, consent could be implicit. For example, if a person receives, completes and returns a postal questionnaire, the act of completion and return implies consent to participate in the research (provided there has been adequate disclosure, s/he is competent and understands the information, participation is voluntary etc.).

## Confidentiality

The Data Protection Act 1998 states the following requirements.[3]

- Personal data shall be processed fairly and lawfully. This means the individual must be informed about who will control the data, how it will be used and provided with any other relevant information which should be given to the data subject to ensure that process is conducted fairly.
- Personal data should be obtained only for one or more specified and lawful purposes and shall not be further processed in any manner incompatible with the explanation given to patients when the information was collected.
- Personal data shall be adequate, relevant and not excessive in relation to the purpose or purposes for which they are processed. When conducting research, it is tempting to collect as many data variables as possible. However, this increases cost of data collection and data entry, and may affect participation rates if subjects are asked to complete long questionnaires.
- Data should be accurate and, where necessary, kept up to date.
- Appropriate technical and organisational measures should be taken against unauthorised or unlawful processing of personal data and against accidental loss or destruction of, or damage to, personal data. It is important that researchers recognise that what they perceive as abstract numbers or other information may relate to very personal and sensitive facts about a person.
- Personal data should not be kept for longer than is necessary. If research is to be published, then it may be necessary to keep the original data in case the analysis is queried.

---

**Case study stage 4**

**Collecting and analysing the research data**

Ethical approval was sought from the LREC for this study. Study practices were recruited from a list of randomly selected practices. Out of ten practices approached, seven agreed to participate. People registered with these practices and having diabetes were identified from practice prescribing information and practice diabetes registers. Three different methods of data collection were employed to collect the explanatory and outcome variables of interest.

- Clinical information and details of health service use were collected from the general practice patient records of all participants.
- Postal questionnaires were also sent to all members of the cohort to collect information directly from them about their circumstances and to validate the information from records.
- Routine hospital data on admissions were also collected and compared with the information from records and questionnaires.

---

# Learning objective 7: undertaking appropriate data collection and analysis to address a specific research question

Once the protocol has been written, and ideally peer-reviewed, and funding and ethical approval obtained if needed, you can start to recruit participants (if appropriate) and to collect your research data. At this point unanticipated problems often arise. This is why a pilot phase is always worth considering, and why study protocols may need to be adapted after the study has started if circumstances change or new information becomes available.

---

**Exercise 9.4**

Consider the research questions addressed in the case study.

- What data would you choose to collect to answer the research question?
- How would you then analyse it?
- What ethical or confidentiality issues would arise?

---

**Case study stage 5**

**Disseminating the research findings**

The main finding from this study was that those people with diabetes who attended hospital diabetes clinics were admitted to hospital less often. The study also showed that access to a car was a significant determinant of attending a hospital clinic. No such associations were found in relation to routine reviews in primary care. Once the study was complete, the results were presented to local stakeholders in diabetes services (service commissioners, service providers, clinicians and people with diabetes) and the interpretation and significance of the results discussed. A summary of results was sent to the research participants and they were also asked whether they had any comments on the findings. The results were presented at conferences and published in specialist and general medical journals.[4–7]

---

## *Avenues for disseminating the research findings*

The main avenues for trying to ensure that research findings will increase understanding of the research topic and, if appropriate, will be used to change policy and practice are:

- talks, workshops and seminars
- conference posters and presentations
- published reports
- research papers in peer-reviewed journals
- formal meetings and informal discussions of findings with colleagues, practitioners or policy-makers.

Other ways of getting research findings into practice include using academic detailing (one-to-one meetings with practitioners), and the use of evidence-based clinical guidelines is discussed elsewhere in this book (*see* Chapter 3).

# Learning objective 8: understanding how to interpret research findings and how to use them to improve health

Just as you need to critically appraise other people's research papers and consider how any weaknesses of their methods may affect interpretation of their findings, you need to discuss your own findings critically. There are a number of useful published guides to critical appraisal of medical literature in both books and journals that provide checklists of issues to consider. 'Evidence-based public health' draws on a wider range of research than evidence-based medicine, but many of the principles in using research findings appropriately are the same. It is still important to critically evaluate the strength and weakness of any research evidence you use (*see* further reading on critical appraisal). It is particularly important to consider whether research findings in a specific population are likely to be directly applicable to your own population, as many public health interventions need to be adapted appropriately for a particular setting or population.

# Further exercises

The boxes give three research topics for you to consider. There may be scope to collate and use the findings of previous research and to conduct further research in all these areas. Choose one of these topics or one arising from your own practice and develop an answerable research question. Do a literature search before designing a study that could answer your research question.

---

**Exercise 9.5**

**Epidemiological research**

There is concern about the potential health effects of increasing use of mobile phones in the local population. It is suggested that 'research is urgently needed' to address the issue.

- What is the main research question? Suggest appropriate study designs that would address the need to provide evidence-based advice in a relatively short time.

---

**Exercise 9.6**

**Health services research**

It has been shown by analyses of routine information that people living in more deprived areas are less likely to have coronary bypass surgery, although it is also known that they have a relatively high rate of cardiovascular mortality. In order to develop interventions to improve appropriate access you need to understand why.

- What hypotheses might you wish to test? Frame some specific research questions. What research methods would be appropriate to answer these questions?

---

**Exercise 9.7**

**Evaluating interventions**

Local mortality rates for smoking-related diseases are high. Reducing smoking rates is a local priority and so a programme of smoking cessation interventions is proposed.

- What should be done? How can the programme results be evaluated?

---

# References

1 Pope C and Mays N (1995) Reaching the parts other methods cannot reach: an introduction to qualitative methods in health and health services research. *BMJ.* **311**: 42–5.

2 Gillick V (1994) Confidentiality, contraception and young people. *BMJ.* **308**: 342–3.

3 Mullock J and Leigh-Pollitt P (2000) *The Data Protection Act Explained* (2e). The Stationery Office, London.

## Results of the research case study

4 Goyder EC, McNally PG, Drucquer M, Spiers N and Botha JL (1998) Shifting of care for diabetes from secondary to primary care, 1990–95: review of general practices. *BMJ.* **316**:1505–6.

5 Goyder EC, Spiers N, Botha JL, McNally P and Drucquer M (1999) Do diabetes clinic attendees stay out of hospital? A matched case-control study. *Diabetic Medicine.* **16**: 687–91.

6 Goyder EC, Botha JL and McNally P (2000) Inequality in access to routine care for diabetes: evidence from an historical cohort study. *Quality in Health Care.* **9**: 85–9.

7 Goyder EC and Botha JL (2001) Characteristics of non-responders to service use questionnaires. *Public Health.* **115**: 78–9.

# Further reading

## On using other people's research

- Sackett DL *et al.* (2000) *Evidence-based Medicine: how to practice and teach EBM* (2e). Churchill Livingstone, Edinburgh.

## Critical appraisal of primary research

- Greenhalgh T (1997) How to read a paper: assessing the methodological quality of published papers. *BMJ.* **315**: 305–8.
- *Online tutorial*: www.shef.ac.uk/~scharr/ir/mschi/unit4/index.htm.

## Critical appraisal of secondary research

- Greenhalgh T (1997) How to read a paper: papers that summarise other papers (systematic reviews and meta-analyses). *BMJ.* **315**: 672–5.
- Oxman AD, Cook DJ and Guyatt GH (1994) Users' guides to the medical literature, VI. How to use an overview. Evidence-Based Medicine Working Party. *JAMA.* **272**(17): 1367–71.
- *Online tutorial*: www.shef.ac.uk/~scharr/ir/mschi/unit5/index.htm.

## How to do a systematic review

- Chalmers I and Altman DG (1995) *Systematic Reviews.* BMJ Publishing Group, London.
- Cochrane Collaboration (1996) *The Cochrane Library* (database on disk and CD-ROM). The Cochrane Collaboration and Update Software, Oxford.
- Mulrow CD and Oxman AD (eds) (1994) Section VI: preparing and maintaining systematic reviews. In: *The Cochrane Collaboration Handbook.* Cochrane Collaboration, Oxford.
- NHS Centre for Reviews and Dissemination (1996) *Undertaking Systematic Reviews of Research on Effectiveness: CRD guidelines for those carrying out or commissioning reviews* (CRD Report No. 4). NHS Centre for R&D, York.
- *Online tutorial available*: www.shef.ac.uk/uni/academic/R-Z/scharr/triage/docs/systematic/index.htm.

## Doing your own research

- Bowling A (1995) *Measuring Disease: a review of disease-specific quality of life measurement scales.* Open University Press, Buckingham.
- Bowling A (1997) *Measuring Health: a review of quality of life measures* (2e). Open University Press, Buckingham.
- Hennekens CH and Buring JE (1987) Epidemiological study design: cross-sectional, cohort and case-control methods. In: CH Hennekens, JE Buring and SL Mayrent (eds) *Epidemiology in Medicine.* Little, Brown and Co, Boston, MA.
- Jackson CJ and Furnham A (2000) *Designing and Analysing Questionnaires and Surveys: a manual for health professionals and administrators.* Whurr Publishers Ltd, London.

### Randomised controlled trials

- Jadad AR (1998) *Randomised Controlled Trials: a user's guide.* BMJ Books, London.

## Health services research

- Black N, Brazier J, Fitzpatrick R and Reeves B (1998) *Health Services Research Methods: a guide to best practice.* BMJ Books, London.
- Crombie IK and Davies HTO (1996) *Research in Health Care: design, conduct and interpretation of health services research.* Wiley, Chichester.
- Fulop N, Allen P, Clarke A and Black N (2001) *Studying the Organisation and Delivery of Health Services: research methods.* Routledge, London.

## Qualitative methods

- Krueger R (1994) *Focus Groups: a practical guide for applied research* (2e). Sage Publications, Thousand Oaks, CA.
- Mays N and Pope C (eds) (1996) *Qualitative Research in Health Care.* BMJ Publishing Group, London.

# Dissemination

- Hall GM (1998) *How to Write a Paper.* BMJ Books, London.

# Ethics

- Beauchamp TL and Childress JF (2001) *Principles of Biomedical Ethics* (5e). Oxford University Press, New York.

# CHAPTER 10

# A day in the life of a public health practitioner: ethically managing self, people and resources

## Ian Welborn

## Introduction

Managing self, people and resources are skills that underpin much of the work of the public health practitioner. There will inevitably be overlaps with the content of the previous chapters, in particular strategic leadership for health (*see* Chapter 8) and collaborative working for health (*see* Chapter 4). To avoid duplication some sections will refer back to those areas explored earlier in the book.

To provide a coherent overview of this topic, I present it as four separate but inter-related sections: stakeholder management; team development and management; project planning and implementation; and self-management – *see* Figure 10.1.

## Learning objectives

The overall aim is to identify some key principles on each of the aforementioned topic areas and highlight some key skills that the public health practitioner will require and need to develop. At different points throughout the chapter, I direct the reader to different aspects of the further reading section for additional exploration.

By working through the contents of this chapter, the reader should:

- be able to understand the basic principles involved in identifying and influencing one's stakeholders, particularly through:
  - acquiring resources
  - getting them 'on board' with any changes that are taking place
  - maintaining their support throughout these changes

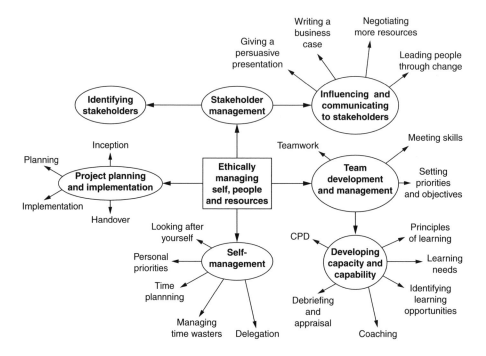

**Figure 10.1:** Structure of the chapter.

- be able to understand the key stages in setting up, planning, implementing and handing over a project
- be able to recognise the key features for:
  - effective teamworking
  - setting clear priorities and objectives
  - running effective team meetings
  - developing the capacity and capability of the whole team and its individual members
- be able to understand the key principles in effectively managing themselves through:
  - setting personal priorities
  - managing time wasters
  - effective delegation
  - personal development planning.

Start by reading the case study and then answering the questions posed. Check your answers by reading the notes in the remainder of the chapter.

**Case study**

It is the end of another busy and sometimes difficult day but not untypical for these times. I am sitting in my favourite armchair, reflecting on the ups and downs of the day.

The day had started, as it always does, with a review of my whiteboard. I have found my whiteboard is the best way to manage my work programme. It provides a fast visual overview of priority tasks. I update it each morning and it provides me with my work plan for the day.

This was immediately followed by a multidisciplinary meeting on hepatitis B screening and antenatal services. This was not a good start to the day as these meetings, which have now been running for a couple of months, always end up with the consultant microbiologist and myself having some sort of head-to-head argument. The project had started well. I had been asked to set up the group, which includes midwives and genito-urinary staff as well as this consultant microbiologist. We started work by developing a care pathway and up to this point we were all working well together. However, when we started to discuss antenatal screening, things between us began to deteriorate. I had suggested we should put delivery of this service up for tender between local provision by the consultant microbiologist's department or by using the National Blood Service. This suggestion certainly upset him but the real arguments came when we started to discuss what we would do if the results of the screening were positive. I wanted to appoint an antenatal co-ordinator who would inform all concerned, follow up on contacts and generally manage this process. The consultant microbiologist, on the other hand, felt that the only person who should be informed was the person who referred the individual and that it would be up to this individual to manage things from this point. There is something about this consultant that makes my blood boil. I am not normally an aggressive person but his arrogant behaviour brings out the worst in me. As, recently, the meetings are poorly attended, the others obviously are not happy with the way things are going. I must find some way of trying to resolve this problem!

Then followed a meeting with my trainee – a regular fortnightly review of my trainee's projects and her development needs. I had assigned her a particularly challenging project on colon cancer. The five-year survival rate was significantly lower than in other districts. However, it has been a difficult project as the figures were built up from two regions and the reporting of cancer and survival rates was inaccurate. This has disguised a poor service although by the time the trainee was looking into this, improvement measures had already been put in place. I felt that this project had a number of advantages for the trainee. It was a good learning opportunity providing good experience in epidemiology, a recognised development need; it will give her the basis for a publication and raise her profile to meet her future career prospects. Unfortunately, there had been little progress on the project; the reason being given was the pressures of other work. However, I suspect that there was a lack of motivation for the project and so I spent most of the time exploring the reasons for this and finding ways to remotivate her. As part of this process I found she was struggling to understand some of the statistical aspects of the project and I took some time to coach the trainee through this particular problem. In the end, I was very happy with the outcome of the session and I believe the trainee was too.

My next appointment was with a curtain chord. It was my privilege to open the curtains on a plaque commemorating the opening of a new stroke rehabilitation unit. This has been a success story. The stroke mortality levels were higher locally than in the rest of the country. It had been looked at on a previous occasion and a stroke rehabilitation unit was planned but finally 'knocked on the head' due to a lack of funding. Since then there has been much more evidence that stroke rehabilitation units work and finally we have a consultant who is committed and prepared to champion it. However, the way forward was not without its problems. The consultant had stubbornly wanted to 'cherry-pick' the patients who would most benefit from the unit, whereas the evidence shows that all patients will benefit. In the end, after a lot of discussion, the consultant came around to my way of thinking. It started off well. We had a good team of committed people with representatives from acute and community units and patient user groups. Working around a care pathway, we developed a strategy but then hit the same problem as before – no funding. However, the difference in this case was that we had set up a meeting to generate ideas and develop an action plan to get the stroke rehabilitation unit back on the priority list. We mobilised a lot of support, which eventually produced the successful outcome. I had much pleasure and satisfaction from opening the unit today.

The remainder of the day, I spent in my office producing reports, answering emails and dealing with various phone calls. I had hoped to leave on time this evening but, as usual, I seemed to get bogged down with trivia. That meant this report, which had to be completed today, was written up when others had gone home so there were no interruptions to distract me. I wonder why I invariably end up doing these sorts of last-minute-panic report-writing sessions? It is probably because I take on too much; my time gets taken up going to meetings I know will be a waste of time and I end up doing work myself which others in the project group should be sharing, if they were more committed or had more time. This report is a typical example. It is about extending breast screening. It is a difficult problem that no one thinks is important or feasible. This means we end up having the wrong people at the meetings so nothing can get decided, we lack information to make appropriate decisions and no one is prepared or able to progress the work. In the end, nothing gets done unless I am the one doing it.

Actually, taking some time out to reflect like this on the day has been useful as it has highlighted some lessons I need to learn about doing things differently if I am going to be more effective in my job.

Before reading the remainder of the chapter, answer the following questions on the case study.

Exercise 10.1

1 What possible factors could have contributed to the conflict between the public health practitioner and the consultant microbiologist?
2 How can the public health practitioner resolve the conflict between him and the consultant microbiologist? How could this conflict have been avoided in the first place?
3 What action should the public health practitioner take to manage the team involved with the antenatal screening project?
4 How would you approach the interview for remotivating the trainee? What factors would you take into account in determining your approach?
5 What steps would you take to identify the original training needs of the trainee?
6 How could you set up this learning opportunity for the trainee in such a way that she would be motivated from the start?
7 How would you coach the trainee through the statistical problem she was having?
8 What are the possible factors that made the stroke rehabilitation unit project successful?
9 How do you think the public health practitioner could approach the consultant in order for him to drop his 'cherry-picking' idea?
10 What possible steps might the project group take to gain the necessary support to raise the priority and gain the necessary funding for the stroke rehabilitation unit?
11 What does the public health practitioner need to do to use his/her time more effectively?
12 What might be some of the personal features of the public health practitioner that contributed to the ineffective use of time?
13 Think of some of the main time wasters you have to deal with. What steps do you take to manage these and what more could you do?
14 What should the public health practitioner now do to ensure s/he improves the way s/he works?

# Stakeholder management

## Identifying your stakeholders

In the case study presented here, the success or otherwise of the projects depended upon the public health practitioner gaining the support of the stakeholders involved. *Stakeholders* are any individuals or groups of individuals who have some interest in the project or programme. Such stakeholders are likely to include people both inside and outside of your organisation: those directly involved in the project and those who are seen to have a marginal interest.

Stakeholders can be categorised into three broad types.

- Those who *care* – people who have an interest in the outcome of a project usually because it has some impact upon them as individuals. This impact may be some gain or loss or in some way affects their feelings, values or beliefs.
- Those who *know* – people who have an interest in the project in terms of providing (or withholding) information, knowledge or technical expertise.
- Those who *can* – people who have the power and influence to either support the project and ensure its success, or hinder or block its progress.

Some stakeholders will fall into more than one category.

With the hepatitis B screening project, the consultant microbiologist was a key stakeholder who was handled badly and as a result blocked the way forward for the public health practitioner. On the other hand, the consultant involved in the stroke rehabilitation unit was handled well, even though he was a difficult person, and as such supported the public health practitioner's way of developing the project. Both were key stakeholders *who care, know and can.* Therefore, a key factor in the long-term success of any project depends to a great extent on how well you manage your key stakeholders.

First, identify the key stakeholders, i.e. those who have the greatest impact on the success or failure of your project, and categorise them as those who *care, know* or *can.* Although you must not entirely ignore the other stakeholders, your main energies need to be concentrated on those with the greatest impact, whether positive or negative. Don't fall into the trap of only concentrating on those who have a negative attitude. Always nurture and look after your allies to maintain their positivity.

- For those who *care,* identify what they would like to see or not like to see as a successful outcome from the project (their success criteria). Then draw up a *communications plan* for the whole of the project to ensure they feel comfortable that progress is being made in line with their success criteria.
- For those who *know,* identify their contribution to the project and involve them in the planning process as much as possible.
- For those who *can,* draw up a *commitment plan* by identifying their existing level of commitment to the project or programme and the minimum level of commitment needed for it to be successful.[1] For those where there are gaps between these two positions, develop an action plan for increasing and maintaining their commitment.

For some, this level of caution and planning might seem unnecessary and peripheral to 'getting the job done'. However, it does not matter how beneficial, how well organised, how well planned or how well designed and developed a project is, without the acceptance and support of your key stakeholders it will fail. Briner *et al.* deal with this process of stakeholder analysis in more depth.[2]

# Influencing and communicating to stakeholders

In managing your stakeholders, identifying whom you need on your side is only half the battle. The other half is having effective communications and influencing skills to bring them over to your way of thinking and keep them 'on board'. There is a wide range of situations where the public health practitioner is required to apply such influencing techniques.

- *Giving a persuasive presentation*: this involves analysing your audience, having an appropriate structure for your presentation to meet your aims, developing clear and attention-grabbing visual aids and acquiring good platform skills. To explore this topic in more depth, *see* the 'presentation skills' section of further reading.
- *Writing a business case*: analysing your readership and having an appropriate structure are equally important in this situation. Writing in a clear, concise and positive style is also important. To explore this topic in more depth, *see* Chapter 6 and the 'effective writing skills' section of further reading.
- *Negotiating for more resources*: whether this is for more money, staff or other facilities, the public health practitioner will need to develop such negotiating skills as the more traditional positional bargaining approach and the more collaborative 'principled negotiation' recently developed by Fisher and Ury.[3] To explore this topic in more depth, *see* the 'negotiating skills' section of further reading.
- *Leading people through change*: understanding an individual's reaction to change and the causes of resistance are important factors in determining strategies for the managing of people through change and gaining their commitment to it. To explore this topic in more depth, *see* the 'managing change' section of further reading.

## *Principles of effective influencing*

Throughout your reading of these topics you will become aware of a wide range of influencing techniques available to the public health practitioner. However, there are some basic principles that apply in all of these.

- *Good preparation*: essential in all forms of influencing, the more time that is given over to effective preparation, the greater the chance of success is likely to be in influencing the situation. Such factors that need to be considered in this preparation stage include the following.

- *Identify your own needs, objectives and values* – enables greater flexibility of approach.
- *Establish your power base* – in any influencing situation, your success will depend to a great extent upon your ability to establish an adequate power base. Such power may come from a range of sources such as:
  (i)   the authority of your role in the organisation
  (ii)  your expertise
  (iii) your access to resources
  (iv)  your networks
  (v)   your personal presence and integrity.
  If your power base is low, you will need to find ways of building this up prior to entering any influencing situation.
- *Understand issues, political context, vested interests* – understanding the broader political context within which you are working is vital to your ability to influence a situation.

- *Gain understanding of others' needs and goals*: if these are not known to you beforehand, you need to establish them as quickly as possible once in the influencing situation.
- *Establish credibility and trust*: *credibility* comes from your power base whereas *trust* comes from demonstrating that you fully appreciate and value the other parties' points of view and do nothing to diminish them in the process of influencing them. If there is a history of poor trust in the past, then more will have to be done to regain this trust prior to the process of influencing the other parties.
- *Manage your own feelings*: there is a greater chance of a positive and construct-ive outcome being achieved by taking an assertive approach. This is where the strength of your feelings are expressed, while keeping your emotions in check.
- *Be sensitive/aware of others' feelings*: others feel as equally strongly about their point of view as you do and may not be able to keep their own feelings in check. Do not get hooked into any destructive behaviour just because the other party does.
- *Get agreement on the problem*: most parties define their wants in an influencing situation in terms of a solution to a problem they have. It is much easier to reach a satisfactory outcome to the situation if there is agreement about the problem in terms of the needs and concerns of all parties involved.
- *Be flexible, adaptable and creative about solutions*: seek the win–win solution. Only look at solutions once there has been agreement about the problem as defined by all parties concerned. People are much more prepared to explore other solutions if they know their needs are being taken into consideration.

Always present such solutions in terms of how they will meet the other's needs and be prepared to be flexible and look for creative solutions that meet everyone's needs.

*   *Develop an alternative to an agreed outcome*: always have a 'backstop' to an agreed solution. It will not always be possible to find a win–win solution but there are usually other ways of achieving your needs. Having these in reserve will strengthen your position. Even if you do not win this issue, you can always use it for gaining something in the future or for building a stronger relationship with the other parties.

If we now look back at the case study, we can see that the public health practitioner had not kept his/her feelings in check in communicating with the consultant microbiologist. This probably prevented him/her from being prepared to listen to the microbiologist and therefore s/he did not take this person's needs into account in looking for a solution to the problem. On the other hand, there was much more respect for the consultant involved with the development of the stroke rehabilitation unit even though he was a difficult character. This, together with the research evidence supporting the public health practitioner's point of view, which comes from good preparation, probably allowed for much greater mutual understanding in the discussion and achievement of an acceptable outcome.

To explore this topic in more depth, *see* the 'power and influence', 'conflict management' and 'handling difficult people' sections of further reading.

# Project planning and implementation

As can be seen from the case study, much of the work of the public health practitioner involves projects, whether it is the development of a service, the establishment of a smoking cessation policy or an outbreak investigation. All projects have a beginning, middle and an end and often result in some form of change to behaviour, working practices, systems, etc. Being an effective project manager is, therefore, a vital skill for the public health practitioner. Although stakeholder management and team management (dealt with later in the chapter) are key elements of project management, a third element is the management of the project life-cycle – i.e. guiding the project through its four stages of inception, planning, implementation and handover.

## Inception stage

Once a project has been conceived, the first and probably most important phase of the project is to develop a clear and agreed definition of the project, a *project synopsis.*

There are a number of processes that may need to take place as part of the development of the synopsis – although, depending upon the type and size of the project, some of these processes may be unnecessary or less important.

- *Establish the feasibility of the project.*
- *Set up the project team* by getting the right membership and establishing effective ways of working.
- *Develop an agreed vision* with the project sponsor and the members of the project team about what the future will look like after the change has taken place.
- *Develop a shared understanding of the 'present situation'* and the need for change. Useful analytical techniques such as *relationship diagrams*,[4] *multiple cause diagrams*,[4] *fishbone (cause and effect) analysis*[5] and *SWOT Analysis*[6] can be helpful here.
- *Set clear and specific objectives.*
- *Define success criteria* as standards by which success in the project will be judged as well as the constraints of such things as time and money that will limit what can be achieved.
- *Identify barriers to success*: a useful technique for analysing such barriers is *force field analysis.*[7]
- *Explore and select the best strategic option* or solution to the problem, against the agreed success criteria and constraints.
- *Establish a commitment to resources*: by this stage you may not know exactly what resources will be required but the overall strategy selected may give you an idea of a 'ballpark figure' in terms of financial, material and human resources. It is useful to ensure you have got an overall commitment to this level of resource requirement before a project synopsis is finally agreed.

From these processes it is possible to develop a project synopsis, with the project sponsor or steering group, in conjunction with the project leader, normally drawing up the terms of reference. Such a synopsis must include:

- the reasons for the project
- the required outputs and quality
- success criteria and constraints
- outline of the broad strategy
- project hierarchy – it is important for all involved to understand how the project is to be controlled.

Once you feel you have a clear contract and mandate for the project, you can move into the planning phase.

## Planning stage

In order to carry out the detailed planning of the project, the following steps are required.

- *Identify the tasks*: these will be tasks concerned with the running and administration of the project as well as those involved in the actual work content.
- *Order the tasks*: separate out the tasks into a logical sequence (e.g. a flow diagram). For simple projects produce a *Gantt chart*.[8] This does not show dependencies but is a useful time-planning tool. For more complex and time-dependent projects, networking techniques such as a *critical path analysis* are needed.
- *Allocate resources*: by using the Gantt chart as a base, examine each activity group, decide who is to be involved and their responsibilities. Then identify the resources needed and allocate these to each activity group.
- *Estimate time* requirements, particularly where this is a critical factor.
- *Contingency planning*: however effective your planning process, there will always be other factors conspiring to prevent implementation going to plan. Many of these problems can be foreseen with a little forethought and contingency plans drawn up to deal with them.

## Implementation stage

If the planning process is carried out well, implementation is the enactment of that plan. However, in reality, things do not always go according to plan and it is important to respond flexibly to situations as they arise rather than sticking rigidly to the plan. Therefore, in practice, an effective project team constantly reviews the situation against the project synopsis and modifies as appropriate. This involves testing out changes with the stakeholders, identifying any problems, replanning where necessary and renegotiating resources and support if required. In effect, the implementation phase is a series of continuous 'plan–do–review' cycles.

- *Managing the transition*: where projects involve major change, such projects flounder at this stage because they do not take into account the human factors involved in implementing change. The effective management of this transitional process is vital if the project is to be implemented according to the plan.
- *Monitoring the project and reporting progress*: not every element of the project is crucial to its success, and regular review meetings (say every week) may result in some problems remaining unresolved until the next meeting. Instead, by identifying critical monitoring points, potential problems can be dealt with early. It is important for the monitoring system to be effective but not become unwieldy or an end in itself. Therefore, selection of the appropriate

method depends on balancing the level of risk and trust, and the level of bureaucracy and administrative load created.

- *Taking corrective action*: when your project hits a snag, as it almost certainly will, you will need to analyse what went wrong in order to take corrective action and avoid similar mistakes in the future. The essential factor is to remove any feelings of blame and guilt, which may damage effective working relationships and block the resolution of the problem. It is important to separate out responsibility and blame. Instead, by taking a clear problem-solving approach to working out what went wrong, why and what the implications are, corrective action can be effected.

## Handover stage

By definition, the project must have an end point. If the project has been successful then it is now time to hand over the management for full integration into the normal processes of the organisation.

- *Project closedown*: project closedown is not always a simple process. There are various reasons the project may continue beyond its end point. To avoid this, there should be a clear signing-off point, an agreed handover process and agreed follow-up support.
- *Review of project*: it is vital there is a full review of the project to gain maximum learning from the process to improve future performance.
- *Celebration of success and dismantling of the team*: it is important that all team members celebrate their successes and signal the emotional disconnection from the team.

In the case study, two of the projects, hepatitis B screening and the stroke rehabilitation unit, developed care pathways, which provided a vision and structure from which to work. It is not clear, from the information available, how much of the project planning structure outlined above was followed but most of the problems seem to lie with the skills of influencing rather than the process. This was not the case for the other two projects described.

In the case of the trainee's project, it seems that a project synopsis was not fully drawn up as the scope of the project changed and the project sponsor, the public health practitioner, had not got the project leader, the trainee, fully on board. With the breast screening extension, there was no feasibility study carried out, and no clear vision or realistic goals set that people were prepared to commit to. As a result, the wrong people were selected for the project team. As such, they were not prepared to commit their time to the project. The inception stage is often the most vital in ensuring the success of a project and the one that is the most overlooked. To explore this topic in more depth, *see* the 'project management' and 'managing change' sections of further reading.

# Team development and management

Most organisational outcomes are achieved through teams working effectively both while they are together as a group and when they are working apart. The public health practitioner will often work in teams to achieve results. A *team* can be defined as 'any group of people who must significantly relate with each other in order to accomplish shared objectives'. Such teams can be permanent or temporary, functional or multidisciplinary, within a single organisation or multi-agency. Nevertheless, each group is unique as it is the combination of the individuals involved that changes its dynamics. There are, however, some basic principles that, if followed, can provide insight into these dynamics and improve the effectiveness in the way the team works.

## Effective teamwork

Some teams seem to work well together whereas other teams seem to have real difficulties in achieving anything. For any team to be effective in achieving its stated goals it needs to have the following six elements well developed (*see* Figure 10.2).[9]

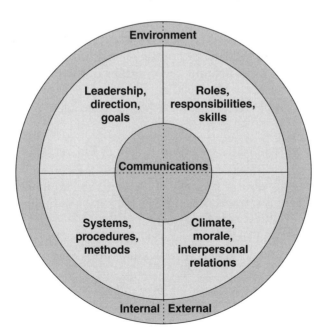

**Figure 10.2:**   Elements of an effective working team.

## 1 Leadership, direction, goals

Keeping the team's commitment and performance high throughout a project is a vital aspect of leadership. Leadership has been dealt with in more detail in Chapter 8, but there are some specific factors that need to be highlighted here.

- The role of the leader must be clear and accepted.
- The leader's style in terms of the level of supervision/delegation and support must be appropriate to the team membership.
- The leader must be able to maintain control and discipline.
- The leader must have a clear vision of what is to be achieved and be able to communicate this to other team members.
- The leader must maintain enthusiasm and commitment throughout the project by constantly highlighting priorities, keeping in touch, and being available to discuss problems and provide support.
- The leader must interface with the rest of the organisation to 'pave the way' for team members.
- Leadership can change between members in the group to meets the needs of the project/group.
- The team must work towards a shared vision and specific and measurable goals.

*Setting high performance objectives*: a particularly important skill in providing direction and harnessing the energies of the team is through the ability to set high performance objectives around key priorities of the job. Establishing key priorities is dealt with later in the chapter under 'Self-management'.

To be effective as an objective setter, the leader needs to adopt certain principles. Objectives need to be SCRAMMARS:[10]

- *Specific*: describing what it is you want to achieve in very clear and precise terms.
- *Challenging*: stretching but achievable, if they are to maximise potential.
- *Resourced*: sufficient resources must be made available if the objectives are to be accomplished to the standards required.
- *Aligned*: all objectives need to be compatible with those of other people within the team or organisation, otherwise individuals and departments will tend to work against each other.
- *Measurable*: quantifiable targets or performance standards and, where this is not possible, qualitative objectives.
- *Monitored*: control systems need to be developed which monitor progress against these objectives.
- *Agreed*: individuals need to accept and agree their objectives if they are to be committed to them.

- *Relevant*: objectives should be regularly reviewed and amended where irrelevant or inappropriate.
- *Supported*: support may take the form of activities such as representations to other departments, providing extra resources as well as providing advice and encouragement to team members.

Unless these nine principles are followed, then objective setting as a process will become less effective as a mechanism for performance management and review.

## 2 Roles, responsibilities and skills

A second element of an effective team is to have the right membership. This requires clear definition of the roles, responsibilities and skills necessary for the team to achieve its goals.

## 3 Systems, procedures and methods

A third element of effective teams is to establish ways of working, in terms of systems and procedures, that ensure co-ordination of effort between team members. This includes identifying the types of meetings required, the purpose of these meetings, the appropriate membership and ensuring effective management through appropriate use of chairing skills and effective meeting procedures such as agendas, discussion papers, minutes, etc.

## 4 Climate, morale and interpersonal relationships

Another essential element of effective teams is a good team spirit, where there is a positive, constructive and supportive climate.

## 5 Communications

This is the element that binds the others together to make each aspect of the team work. In particular, there needs to be:

- clear communication of the goals
- good systems of communication set up and maintained – linking members and co-ordinating activities
- a depth of communication where there is a willingness to share information, feelings, concerns, and provide feedback, etc., in an assertive manner
- development of effective communication and interpersonal skills by individuals.

## 6 *The environment*

This is the element most often overlooked in considering the effectiveness of a team. No team can exist in isolation; it must live in harmony with the environment within which it exists. This may be the internal environment (e.g. other departments) or external environment (e.g. other agencies, the public, etc.). In particular, it must:

- have goals compatible with other aspects of the organisation
- understand and meet the needs of its stakeholders (internal and external)
- be conscious of broader social responsibilities.

In the case study there were two examples of team members not attending meetings or wishing not to be there. In the example of the hepatitis B project, it was because of the poor working *climate* created by the conflict between the consultant microbiologist and the public health practitioner. Some form of problem-solving technique, such as an *option appraisal*, might have been useful in resolving the conflict as this takes the issue back into the control of the team rather than resting with the two individuals. On the other hand, the lack of commitment in the breast screening project, as we have already seen, was due to a belief that an acceptable outcome was not possible; in other words, this was a *leadership* issue.

The stroke rehabilitation project team demonstrated it was able to work effectively together. There was a good climate where all members respected each other and this enabled them to take a very positive and constructive attitude towards the difficulties of funding that previous groups had failed to overcome. The time and commitment that members subsequently put into the project to achieve the successful outcome was self-evident.

To work effectively with a team is a vital role of the public health practitioner but it involves a lot of skill and experience. Every team is different, as its functioning is influenced by the composition and resulting dynamics of the group. To explore this topic in more depth, *see* the 'teamwork' and 'meetings' sections of further reading.

## Developing the capacity and capability of the team and its individual members

The public health practitioner is as effective as the competency of the team that s/he has around him/her. A key responsibility of all managers of staff is to ensure that they have the capacity and capability to do the job both now and in the future. This means continuously encouraging team members to develop new skills and maintain existing ones in addition to your own personal development.

Therefore, all managers have to be trainers. This applies to all public health practitioners, not just those who are designated trainers. To be an effective trainer requires an understanding of the basic principles of learning.

## The principles of learning

Learning is a continuous process throughout our lives. What varies is what we learn, how we learn it, how efficiently we learn and how well we learn. These processes are dependent upon factors internal to the learner (e.g. personality, needs, intelligence and potential) and the external conditions in which the learning takes place. By understanding the internal factors and managing the external factors, the trainer can do a lot to facilitate the learning process. Some of the key principles of learning are listed below.

1 Learning occurs within the learner and is activated by the learner; all the trainer can do is provide the right conditions for learning to take place.
2 Learning is a co-operative and collaborative process. It would take too long to learn everything by trial and error.
3 Learning is the discovery of the personal meaning and relevance of ideas. For learning to stick, it must be linked to our existing knowledge and committed to our long-term memory.
4 Most learning is a consequence of experience and reflection.
5 Learning is an evolutionary process. Learners have to go through the learning cycle many times before it is fully learned.
6 Learning takes place at different rates. It is not a smooth process; there will be times when the learner feels that s/he is going backwards or not making progress.
7 People vary in terms of how much they can learn at any one time. Learning must be controlled by the pace of the learner.
8 Learning is sometimes a painful process, involving risk and failure.
9 One of the richest resources for learning is the learner him/herself. Often learning to transfer knowledge and skills from one situation to another can be the biggest contribution a trainer can make.
10 The process of learning is emotional as well as intellectual. The learner must take risks and deal with fears when moving into unknown territory.
11 Learning goes through four basic stages before it becomes permanent. Starting with 'unconscious incompetence', the learner moves to 'conscious incompetence' through an increased awareness of personal learning needs, then moves onto 'conscious competence' through a process of learning and coaching and finishes with 'unconscious competence' through practice.
12 Learning should be organised to favour a person's preferred styles of learning.

13 It is important, as a trainer, to create an atmosphere which encourages the learner to take responsibility and ownership of his/her own learning; which recognises people's rights to make mistakes; which tolerates ambiguity; which encourages openness and trust between trainer and learner; and in which people feel accepted and respected.

14 Learners will be more motivated to learn if the following conditions prevail:
- the purpose and goal(s) are clear
- there are high and positive expectations of the learner and the outcome
- tasks are challenging but with a reasonable chance of success
- the learning must be perceived as relevant and meeting the needs of the learner
- there is an acceptable level of risk for both the trainer and the learner
- rewards are clear, valued and attainable by the learner
- there is frequent and regular constructive feedback from the trainer and other respected colleagues
- an appropriate level of support is provided.

Most learning takes place on the job supplemented by more formal training courses, seminars, etc. The training process as outlined in Figure 10.3 tries to represent the various stages in this process. Like all learning processes it is cyclical.

To be an effective trainer, there are some core elements of this process that the trainer needs to carry out effectively.

## Identifying learning needs and establishing a learning contract and training plan

This involves the following procedures.

- Carrying out a review of the learner's previous experience/training and agreeing where certain levels of competence have been achieved and where there are gaps in competence.
- Identifying and agreeing priorities for training based upon identified gaps in competence. They should be defined as a list of learning objectives.
- If possible, producing an agreed outline training plan for the next phase of development, identifying the type of work to be undertaken and discussing the basis upon which assignments will be selected.
- Agreeing with the learner how s/he should collect evidence of competency in each area of training need and emphasising that it is the learner's role to take responsibility for demonstrating s/he has acquired certain levels of competence in the areas where training needs have been identified.

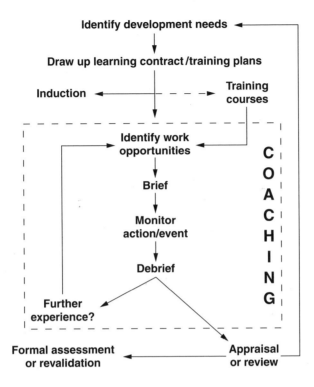

**Figure 10.3:** The training process.[11]

- Agreeing arrangements for reviewing and monitoring progress. In particular, discussing and agreeing how work and learning should be documented by the learner (e.g. log book, portfolio of work, etc.).
- Agreeing the general level of supervision and support required.
- Agreeing the ground rules for feedback.
- Establishing personal terms of reference for your relationship with the learner; in particular, your role as a colleague as well as supervisor and trainer.
- The outcome of these discussions should result in the drawing up of a *learning contract* and *training plan* to reflect the decisions made.

## Selecting and setting up appropriate learning experiences

Using specifically targeted pieces of work that support the learner's learning needs can be one of the most effective ways of developing competence. However, it is important to ensure they are carefully selected and set up. In selecting and setting up an appropriate learning opportunity it is useful to consider the following points.

- Does it suit the learner's preferred learning style?
- Does it have the appropriate level of challenge?
- Does it support the agreed learning objectives?
- Has a task contract or project synopsis been drawn?
- Is the learner motivated to complete the task?
- Has the learner been fully briefed, including the background and political issues surrounding the piece of work?
- Does it add an excessive burden to the learner's workload?

## Coaching learners through problems

From time to time the learners will struggle with some aspects of their work assignments and, if they feel comfortable with their trainer, will approach him/her for help. The trainer has a choice as to whether to help the learners by telling them how to tackle the problem or to help the learners explore the problem and come up with their own solutions. The latter approach is much more effective in developing transferable skills that can be used on similar problems in the future and in building the learners' self-confidence in tackling such problems on their own.

## Debriefing and appraising performance

On completion of a piece of work, or at regular intervals during its progress, the trainer should review the performance of the learner both in terms of the outcomes and in terms of the approach the learner took in tackling the issue. This might be an informal debriefing or a more formal appraisal of a range of projects. In either case the principles are the same – namely, the aim of such a process is developmental and aimed at reviewing and giving the learner feedback on his/her performance, extracting the learning from the experience and identifying future learning needs highlighted by it.

## Encouraging and supporting continuous professional development

Learning is a lifelong process and, whether the member of staff is in a formal training programme or not, all the principles outlined above equally apply if the training process is to be effective. Most professional bodies now have some continuous professional development (CPD) policy and provide encouragement and support to their members. In some cases they require revalidation at regular intervals. This alone is not enough without the additional support of their organisation and their manager.

In the case study, the public health practitioner has implemented many of these aspects. There is a regular and frequent review meeting, projects are selected based upon learning needs and an opportunity for coaching on a difficulty was identified. On the other hand, there was a lack of motivation for the project. As the project was seen to be worthwhile, the lack of interest must have resulted from the inadequate briefing of the project to engage the trainee initially. To explore these topics in more depth, *see* the 'performance management' and 'coaching and training' sections of further reading.

# Self-management

The essential purpose of any job is to achieve results. The role of the public health practitioner is no different in this respect. Such results are achieved by carrying out specific activities to maximise use of the resources at your disposal. For this, you need to have sufficient self-discipline to organise your time and effort effectively. This is what is meant by *self-management.* In addition to the benefits gained by the organisation, the individual also gains as it allows time for other aspects of his/her life outside work.

## Barriers to more effective self-management

The only person that should be blamed for poor self-management is the person him/herself. The roots of the problem invariably rest with the individual who is insufficiently disciplined to manage his/her time. Therefore, if time is to be managed well, you need to take control of your own work time and not allow yourself to be controlled by others or circumstances.

Contributory factors that lead to this lack of self-discipline are:

- an inability to say no
- an inability to plan, preferring action instead
- an inability to prioritise
- a dislike for certain tasks
- an avoidance of decision making
- an avoidance of new tasks
- a need for excessive social contact.

In different ways all these time wasters are ways of maintaining or defending the person's self-esteem and self-confidence and as such are not easily remedied. The first step is for you to recognise which ones stop you from being more self-disciplined. Second, try to be more realistic about the fears which underpin these behaviours by questioning the consequences of not behaving in this way, and finally plan the changes gradually by ensuring the changed behaviour achieves success.

# Managing your time

## Establishing priorities

Effective use of time involves being clear about your priorities and spending your time on those aspects of the job having the greatest effect. The first stage is knowing where your time should be directed by identifying the key result areas of the job and identifying those key tasks core to your role within the organisation. In doing this you will be able to separate out the important from the urgent tasks. The second is to know where your time is actually going by keeping a time log. With both of these sets of information you can then start to decide on the action to take to correct the imbalance.

## Reorganising yourself

Some of the changes you will need to make will be totally under your control. Others will need the agreement or assistance of your boss and your colleagues or possibly people in other departments and even outside the organisation. You will find your time can broadly be divided into two areas: that which *you* control and that which is under the control of *others*. If you want to manage your time, then make sure more of it is under your control!

How you do this is, to a great extent, dependent upon those areas you identified as needing improvement. However, here are some tips to help you organise yourself better.

## Time planning

- Don't use a complex system – it takes time to manage and becomes self-defeating. Develop your own simple 'Time Planning System'.
- Plan *all* your time (including time when you are working on your own). Plan in bold chunks of time.
- Plan three to six months ahead for longer-term goals, e.g. training courses, seminars, etc.
- Allocate time for routine work, known engagements, meetings, etc.
- Don't allocate every hour of the working day to planned activities; allocate a certain amount of time to unplanned activities.
- Review and amend your time plan each week on a rolling three to six monthly basis.
- Plan each day in detail; allow 15 minutes at the beginning of the day or end of the previous day to do this.
- Draw up a 'To Do' list for the day; allocate priorities to each task; review and amend the list each day, changing priorities if necessary.

- Always tackle high-priority tasks first, however large or unpleasant.
- Plan regular meetings for each of your staff individually.
- Plan a time for phone calls.
- Set yourself deadlines on all work and treat them as unbreakable; on large tasks, have intermediate deadlines.

There are many activities within our working life which consume time and take us away from our priority tasks. These time wasters include:

- managing your paperwork (including emails)
- handling both face-to-face and telephone interruptions
- managing your time at meetings that you either attend or chair
- managing your reading time.

There are many techniques for managing these problems. Many of the books listed under the 'time management' section of further reading have many tips for the reader. It is important to select those that suit your style of working if they are to be successful.

## Effective delegation

Whether working with your staff or with others in a multidisciplinary or multi-agency team, it is necessary for the project/team leader to delegate. There is no possibility that the wide range of tasks within his/her responsibility can be handled personally. Thus some responsibilities must be delegated in order to accomplish his/her goals and fulfil his/her role. In addition, it gives more time to tackle strategic issues and plan ahead. Finally, it ensures that the full potential of the staff involved is utilised. This, in turn, encourages motivation and development.

Delegation can be defined as 'giving a subordinate the freedom and authority to handle certain matters on his/her own initiative with the confidence that s/he can do the job successfully'.

This process of delegation involves the following.

- *Giving responsibility*: giving the individual a recognisable element of the organisation's or project's activity in which s/he must make and execute decisions to achieve specified results.
- *Giving authority*: giving the individual permission to control resources and make changes within specified limits so that s/he can achieve the results required of him/her.
- *Retaining control*: ensuring that objectives are achieved by setting clear standards and implementing a process for monitoring progress.
- *Sharing accountability*: making the individual answerable for the consequences of his/her actions, although the ultimate accountability still rests with the manager/project leader.

This is a progressive process that initially takes time in coaching, etc., but will, in the long term, reap benefits.

# Personal development planning

Changing working patterns and working in new areas can feel risky and there is a tendency to withdraw to familiar and comfortable ways of working. To ensure this does not happen, it is important that you set yourself some personal development goals and draw up a personal development plan. Here are some points to consider.

- Only select a few objectives at any one time. Having too many can feel over-whelming and may discourage achievement.
- Ensure these objectives are personally challenging but realistic and achievable.
- Plan exactly what you need to do to achieve these objectives.
- Negotiate the time and other resources necessary to accomplish these objectives.
- Establish a support network that will encourage your achievement of these objectives. This might include your manager, your colleagues, your partner, a mentor, etc.

In the case study, although the public health practitioner used a simple planning tool, the whiteboard, for time planning and prioritisation, there were still problems in time management. This was due to a lack of delegation; an inability to say no; not managing interruptions effectively, possibly as a welcome distraction from doing a difficult or boring report; and attending ineffective meetings without any attempt at either trying to make them more productive or withdrawing from them altogether. To explore this topic in more depth, *see* the 'time management', 'efficient reading' and 'stress management' sections of further reading.

Managing resources, people and self are the core skills that underpin the technical expertise of the public health practitioner. Without denying the importance of the latter, effectiveness is usually dependent upon the successful acquisition of these core skills. They are wide ranging and not easy skills to acquire. In fact, much of the practitioner's development throughout his/her professional life will be in the pursuit of these skills. This chapter has been an attempt to lay down some markers based on some fundamental principles outlined here. However, for the serious student, the attached further reading section will be a key starting point for a more in-depth study of these subjects.

# References

1 Beckhard R and Harris RT (1987) *Organisational Transitions: managing complex change.* Addison-Wesley, Reading, MA.

2 Briner W, Geddes M and Hastings C (1990) *Project Leadership.* Gower, London.

3 Fisher R and Ury W (1983) *Getting to Yes: negotiating agreement without giving in.* Hutchinson, London.

4 Smith R *et al.* (1989) *Planning and Managing Change: course notes.* The Open University Business School, London.

5 Roberts K and Ludvigsen C (1998) *Project Management for Health Care Professionals.* Butterworth-Heinemann, Oxford.

6 Wilson G (1993) *Problem Solving and Decision Making.* Kogan-Page, London.

7 Turrill T (1986) *Change and Innovation: a challenge for the NHS.* The Institute of Health Service Management, London.

8 Bee R and Bee F (1997) *Project Management: the people challenge.* Institute of Personnel and Development, London.

9 Welborn I (1987) *Effective Work Teams.* Workshop handout (unpublished).

10 Welborn I (1988) *Objective Setting.* Workshop handout (unpublished).

11 Welborn I (1995) *The Training Process.* Workshop handout (unpublished).

# Further reading

## Presentation skills

### General

- Caroselli M (1992) *Thinking on Your Feet.* Crisp, Washington, DC.
- Morrisel GL (1984) *Effective Business and Technical Presentations.* Addison-Wesley, Reading, MA.
- Peoples DA (1988) *Presentation Plus.* John Wiley and Sons, Chichester.

### Developing your speaking voice

- Bunch M (1989) *Speak With Confidence.* Kogan-Page, London.

## Effective writing skills

- Goodworth C (1988) *The Secret of Successful Business Letters and Reports.* Heinemann, Portsmouth, NH.
- Sussanne JE (1987) *How to Write Effective Reports.* Gower, London.
- Turk C and Kirkman J (1989) *Effective Writing.* E & FN Spon, London.

## Negotiating skills

- Calaro H and Osram B (1983) *Negotiate for What You Want.* Thorsons, London.

- Kennedy G, Benson J and McMillan J (1985) *Managing Negotiations.* Business Books Paperbacks, London.
- Mills HA (1991) *Negotiate: the art of winning.* Gower, London.

## Power and influence

- Block P (1988) *The Empowered Manager: positive political skills at work.* Jossey-Bass, San Francisco, CA.
- Culbert SA and Donough JJ (1985) *Radical Management: power, politics and the pursuit of trust.* Macmillan, Basingstoke.
- Fisher D and Vilas S (1992) *Power Networking.* Mountain Harbour, Austin, TX.
- Mintzberg H (1983) *Power In and Around Organisations.* Prentice-Hall, London.
- Northstine WL (1989) *Influencing Others.* Crisp, Washington, DC.
- Quick TL (1988) *Power, Influence and Your Effectiveness in Human Resources.* Addison-Wesley, Reading, MA.
- Quick TL (1990) *Mastering the Power of Persuasion.* Executive Enterprises, Philadelphia, PA.
- Srivastva S (1986) *Executive Power.* Jossey-Bass, San Francisco, CA.

## Conflict management

- Kindler HS (1988) *Managing Disagreement Constructively.* Kogan-Page, London.
- Robert M (1982) *Managing Conflict: from the inside out.* University Associates, San Diego, CA.

## Handling difficult people

- Cava R (1990) *Dealing With Difficult People.* Piatkus, London.

## Project management

- Haynes ME (1995) *Project Management.* Kogan-Page, London.
- Klein RL and Ludin IS (1992) *The People Side of Project Management.* Gower, London.
- Lashbrooke G (1991) *A Project Manager's Handbook.* Kogan-Page, London.

## Managing change

- Beckhard R and Harris R (1987) *Organisational Transition: managing complex change.* Addison-Wesley, Reading, MA.

- Kanter RM (1983) *The Change Masters.* Counterpoint, Boulder, CO.
- McLennan R (1989) *Managing Organisational Change.* Prentice-Hall, London.
- Pettigrew A, Ferline E and McKee L (1992) *Shaping Strategic Change.* Sage Publications, Thousand Oaks, CA.
- Plant R (1987) *Managing Change and Making It Stick.* Fontana, London.
- Scott CD and Jaffe DT (1989) *Managing Organisational Change.* Kogan-Page, London.

## Teamwork

- Adair J (1986) *Effective Team Building.* Pan Business/Management, London.
- Chang R, Bader GE and Bloom AE (1995) *Measuring Team Performance.* Kogan-Page, London.
- Francis D and Young D (1979) *Improving Work Groups.* University Associates, San Diego, CA.
- Hastings C, Bixby P and Chawdtry-Lawton R (1986) *Super Teams: blueprint for organisational success.* Fontana/Collins, London.
- Larson CE and Lafesto FMT (1989) *Teamwork: what must go right/what can go wrong.* Sage Publications, Thousand Oaks, CA.
- Woodcock M (1989) *Team Development Manual.* Gower, London.

## Meetings

- Brown P and Hackett F (1990) *Managing Meetings.* Fontana, London.
- Janner G (1986) *Janner on Meetings.* Wildwood House, London.

## Performance management

- Hagemann G (1992) *The Motivation Manual.* Gower, London.
- LeBoeuf M (1986) *How to Motivate People.* Sidgwick and Jackson, London.
- Shaw DG, Schneier CE, Beatty RW and Baird LS (eds) (1995) *The Performance Measurement, Management and Appraisal Sourcebook.* HRD Press, MA.
- Steers RM and Porter LW (1991) *Motivation and Work Behaviour.* McGraw-Hill, Columbus, OH.
- Stewart V and Stewart A (1985) *Managing the Poor Performer.* Gower, London.
- Stewart V and Stewart A (1990) *Practical Performance Appraisal.* Gower, London.

## Coaching and training

- Buckley R and Caple J (1991) *One-to-one Training and Coaching Skills.* Kogan-Page, London.

- Clutterbuck D (1985) *Everyone Needs a Mentor.* Institute of Personnel Management, London.
- Parsloe E (1993) *Coaching, Monitoring and Assessing.* Kogan-Page, London.
- Pedshaw B and Stevens M (1990) *Coaching for Managers.* COIC, Sheffield.

## Time management

- Adair J (1987) *How to Manage Your Time.* Talbot-Adair, Guildford.
- Scott M (1992) *Time Management.* Century Business, London.
- Treacy D (1991) *Clear Your Desk.* Business Books Ltd, London.

## Efficient reading

- Rudd S (1989) *Time Manage Your Reading.* Gower, London.

## Stress management

- Cooper CL, Cooper RD and Eaker LH (1988) *Living with Stress.* Penguin, Harmondsworth.
- Fontana D (1989) *Managing Stress.* BPS and Routledge, London.
- Hatvany I (1996) *Putting Pressure to Work.* Pitman Publishing, London.
- Matheson MT and Ivancevich JM (1987) *Controlling Work Stress.* Jossey-Bass, San Francisco, CA.
- Payne R and Firth-Cozens J (1987) *Stress in Health Professionals.* Wiley, Chichester.

# Index